KU-585-072

# The story of
# **Medicine**
*from papyri to pacemakers*

JUDY LINDSAY

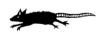

THE BRITISH MUSEUM PRESS

*With thanks to my Dad, himself a doctor,*
*who took some of the photos and appears in the last chapter*

© 2003 Judy Lindsay
First published in 2003 by The British Museum Press
A division of The British Museum Company Limited
46 Bloomsbury Street, London WC1B 3QQ

ISBN 0 7141 3009 5

A catalogue record for this book is available from the British Library.
Designed and typeset in ITC Golden Cockerall by Peter Burgess, Oxford.
Printed and bound in Hong Kong by Paramount Printing Co

► **What we look like inside.**
**A 16-century drawing of**
**a human skeleton leaning**
**on a spade.**

## Illustration Acknowledgements

Photographs are taken by the Photography and Imaging Department of The British Museum and © The Trustees of The British Museum unless otherwise stated.

Ancient Art and Architecture Collection
15 bottom right, 18 bottom left
Tim Beddow/Science Photo Library
27 bottom
Susan Bird 9 bottom, 12 bottom
The British Library 6 left, 7 bottom left,
10 top right, 11 top, 16 bottom, 20 right,
21 bottom right, 22 bottom right, 25
bottom right, 26 top left, 28 top right,
30 top left, 37 bottom left
BSIP VEM/Science Photo Library
37 bottom right
Dr Jeremy Burgess/Science Photo Library
26 bottom and front cover (right)
Peter Burgess, chapter opener drawings
on pages 6, 10, 14, 18, 20, 24, 28, 32, 36, 38
Joyce Filer 24 bottom right
Griffith Institute 21 top left
Ralph Jackson 22 top left
Kings College Hospital NHS Trust
31 top right
Lesley and Roy Adkins Picture Library 15 top
Dr Ken Lindsay 5 bottom, 38 bottom left,
39 top
Mary Evans Picture Library 13 top
National Medical Slide Bank 38 top right
NIBSC/Science Photo Library 31 bottom

Old Operating Theatre 8 bottom.
Richard Parkinson 10  bottom left
The Royal Free Hospital, London front
cover (left)
Richard Revels 21 centre
Françoise Sauze/Science Photo Library
36 bottom right
Science Museum/Science and Society
Picture Library 6 right, 13 bottom left,
23 top (NMPFT/Science & Society Photo
Library), 23 bottom, 24 top right, 25 centre,
26 top right, 30 bottom left (Manchester
Daily Express/Science & Society Photo
Library), 39 bottom right
Dr Linda Stannard, UCT/Science Photo
Library 31 top left
Maximilian Stock/Science Photo Library
13 bottom right
Thackray Medical Museum 17 bottom,
20 bottom left
Tim Vernon, St James University Hospital,
Leeds 37 top left, 39 bottom left
Wellcome Library, London 3, 5 top, 7 top,
7 centre, 8 top, 9 top, 11 bottom right,
12 top, 16 top, 17 top, 19 top right, 22 top
right, 24 left, 27 top left, 27 top right,
29 top left, 29 bottom right, 30 bottom
right, 36 bottom left
York Archaeological Trust Photographic
Unit, photo by Derek Phillips 15
bottom left

ROTHERHAM LIBRARY & INFORMATION SERVICES
J610.9
B48 248 1210
R000500070
SCHOOLS STOCK

# Contents

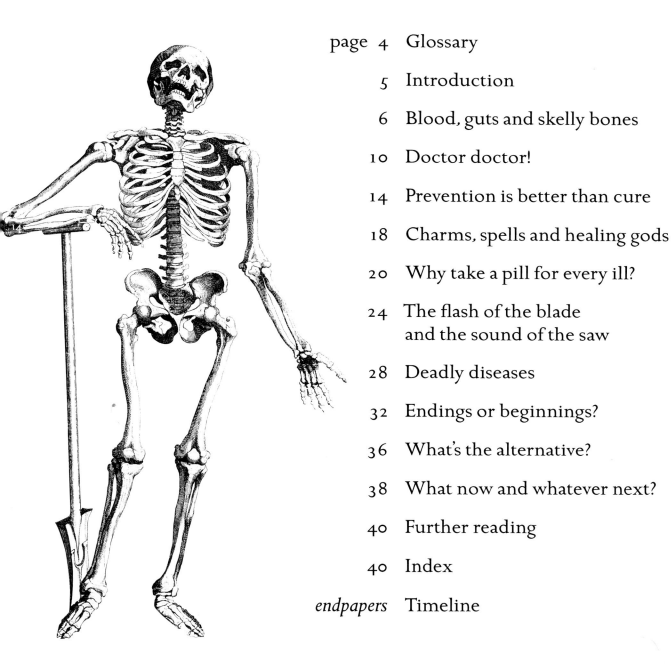

# Glossary

**abscess** a swelling filled with pus

**acupuncture** an ancient Chinese treatment using small needles, inserted into the body at important 'pressure points' to stimulate the nerves

**amulet** a magical charm used to ward off illness

**anaesthetic** something that sends a patient to sleep or numbs a part of the body

**anatomy** the study of what's inside our bodies

**antiseptic** a substance that destroys the harmful micro-organisms that can cause infection

**aqueduct** channels built by the Romans to carry water from one place to another, often incorporating bridges and canals

**Ayurvedic Medicine** classical Indian medical teaching. Ayurveda means 'the knowledge needed for long life'

**bacteria** the group of harmful micro-organisms that cause disease

**bile** bitter fluid produced by the liver

**carbolic acid** antiseptic mixture of chemicals discovered by a German chemist in 1830

**CAT scan** a three-dimensional X-ray

**cauterize** to destroy infected tissue or stop bleeding by burning

**chloroform** colourless, sweet-tasting liquid which causes unconsciousness if inhaled

**diagnosis** identifying a disease from its symptoms

**dissection** the practice of cutting open bodies to see what is inside

**epidemic** a widespread outbreak of disease that affects many people

**ether** colourless liquid used as an anaesthetic

**excrement** waste matter left after food has been digested

**exorcise** to drive away an evil spirit

**genetics** the study of our genes, the blueprints that determine the characteristics of plants and animals

**Hippocratic Oath** an oath, first taken by students of Hippocrates, in which doctors promise they will only use their skills to help patients

**kaolin** fine, soft white clay used in medicines

**massage** stroking, pressing, rubbing or manipulating the body

**micro-organism** an organism so small it can only be seen using a microscope

**organism** living plant or animal

**palaeopathologist** someone who studies prehistoric diseases

**pharmacist** somebody legally qualified to dispense drugs and medicines

**physiology** the study of how our bodies work

**physician** someone legally allowed to be a doctor

**prescription** written instructions from a doctor on what medicines a patient should take

**pustule** pimple or lump filled with pus

**remedy** anything used to cure a disease or illness

**salve** soothing ointment

**shaman** a priest who uses magic to heal the sick

**surgery** treating a patient by cutting, splinting or manipulating the body

**symptom** bodily signs that help a doctor identify what illness a patient is suffering from

**vaccination** deliberately infecting a patient with something fairly harmless to make them immune to a specific disease

**virus** tiny micro-organism that can cause infection

**X-ray** a photograph of the inside of the body

# Introduction

TODAY YOU don't need to be a doctor to know a good deal about your body and how it works. We learn all about the heart, lungs, nerves, arteries and veins in school. We know that we should eat up our greens and drink plenty of milk to get the vitamins and minerals that keep our skin, bones and teeth healthy. You may have taken iron tablets, some cough mixture or an aspirin if you have been feeling a bit under the weather. You probably know what a skeleton looks like, and may even have seen an X-ray of some of your own bones.

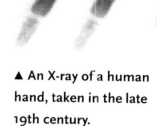

▲ An X-ray of a human hand, taken in the late 19th century.

If you feel sick, you will most likely go and find a useful and reliable adult and tell them what the matter is. If you are snuffly and sneezy and have a sore throat, you will probably be told that you are suffering from a common cold and you should go to bed with a hot-water bottle. If you have cut yourself, then you can be pretty sure that the cut will be washed, then some antiseptic cream and a plaster will do the trick.

If you are too sick to be looked after at home, the useful and reliable adult will take you to a doctor, who knows even more about bodies and how they work. The doctor will try to find out what is wrong with you and give you something to make you better. If the doctor can't do that, you may be sent to a hospital to have special tests or an operation. In the modern world we have become very good at avoiding getting ill and at treating sickness when we do.

But this wasn't always the case. Every civilization has its own healers and its own way of dealing with people who are unwell, but until recently there was a great deal we didn't know about the human body, and that limited what doctors could do to help. Even today people use many different ways of healing – there is no right way or wrong way of making sick people better. The story of how medicine developed is a fascinating journey through many countries over a long period of time.

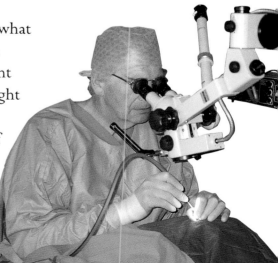

▼ This doctor is examining a patient's ear using an operating microscope.

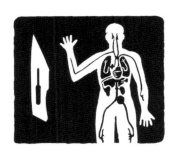

# Blood, guts and skelly bones...
## *Finding out how the body works*

YOU MAY have heard of anatomy and physiology, but do you know what they are? Anatomy is the study of what is inside our bodies. Physiology means finding out how it works. You may also have heard the word dissection, which means cutting a body open to find out more about anatomy and physiology.

### *The mysterious body*

Thousands of years ago people knew very little about these things because most of them had never seen inside a human being. In many cultures dissection was forbidden for religious reasons or because people thought it was disrespectful to cut bodies open: In ancient China only the emperor was allowed to dissect bodies. In India, cutting a dead body with a knife was strictly forbidden, so the only way to study the inside of a body was to store it under water until the skin became soft enough to be poked away with a stick. Just imagine what the body would have looked like!

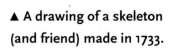

▲ A drawing of a skeleton (and friend) made in 1733.

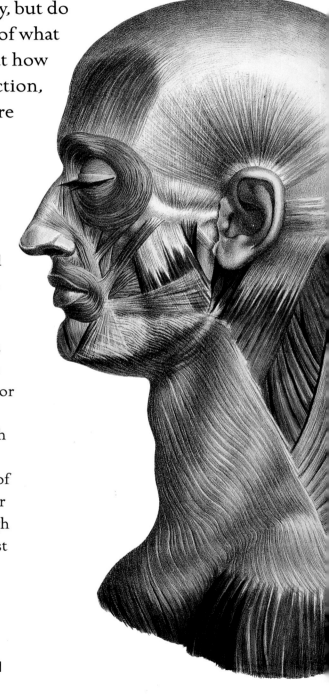

▶ What lies just under your skin: muscles and blood vessels.

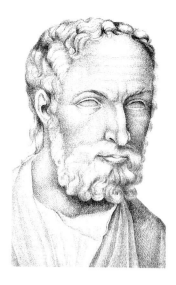

▲ Galen was a Greek doctor who worked for the Romans. He was famous for his anatomical studies.

In the classical world, Greek doctors like Hippocrates (c. 460 – c. 375 BC) and Galen (AD 129 – 216), whose books on anatomy were very famous, almost certainly never dissected a human body. Their knowledge of anatomy was based on animals, which are quite different inside from humans. The result was that for a long time doctors had some strange ideas about how the body works.

Things started to change during the Middle Ages, when Italian doctors at the universities of Padua and Bologna took to dissecting human bodies rather than animals in an attempt to correct some of Galen's mistakes. The first public dissection of a human body took place in Bologna in 1315. However, people still did not like the thought of cutting bodies open, and Italian doctors had to use the bodies of convicted criminals!

▼ Doctors in the 13th century knew how to take a pulse, but they did not know how blood was pumped around the body.

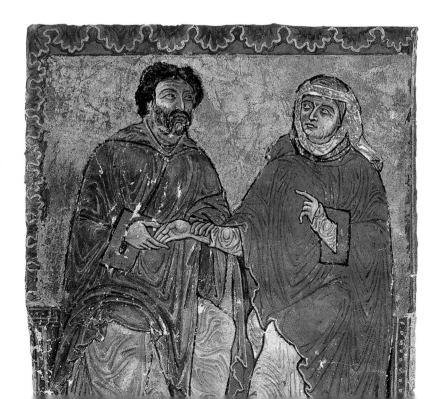

## Bodies in a bedroom

As times moved on, ideas changed. More dissections took place, and people began to find out a great deal more about anatomy and physiology. Then two important discoveries really changed the way we think about the human body. The first was made by Andreas Vesalius (1514 – 64), who was born in Brussels in the Low Countries and received his medical degree from Padua in Italy in 1537.

► Andreas Vesalius published a very famous book on anatomy in 1543.

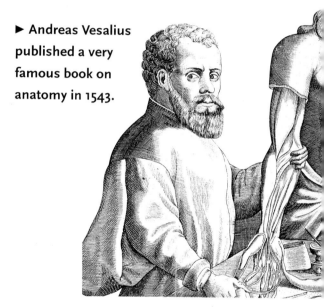

He was determined to find out more about anatomy, and was rumoured to have fought wild dogs for bodies in Italian graveyards. He kept these bodies in his bedroom, where he cut them open and studied them in detail. In 1543 Vesalius published a book based on his studies, with hundreds of illustrations of the inside of the body. The book wasn't quite perfect, but it corrected many of Galen's more obvious mistakes.

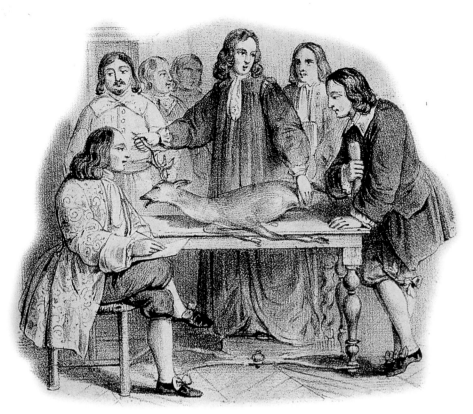

## Digging up the dead

After these discoveries were made people began to realise how important dissection was. However, bodies were still hard to obtain. This led to the rise of a rather gruesome new trade – that of the resurrection men, who went around at night robbing graves so that they could sell the bodies to doctors and medical schools. They roamed around in the dead of night with spades and body bags – it must have been a horrible job. Then, in the early 1800s, two Irishmen went one step further …

## Heart to heart

The second important discovery was made a century later by an Englishman, William Harvey (1578 – 1657). Harvey was a bad-tempered doctor who was obsessed with dissection, and cut open dogs, cats, rats and even snakes! Earlier doctors had only had vague ideas about how the heart pumped blood around the body. Harvey's experiments proved that blood moves from one side of the heart into the lungs, where it absorbs oxygen, and is then pumped back into the heart. Arteries carry blood away from the heart to all the different parts of the body, and the veins carry it back.

▲ Lock up your pets! William Harvey and later doctors would dissect almost anything to find out more about anatomy.

▼ In Victorian times medical students learned about anatomy by watching dissections in operating theatres like this one.

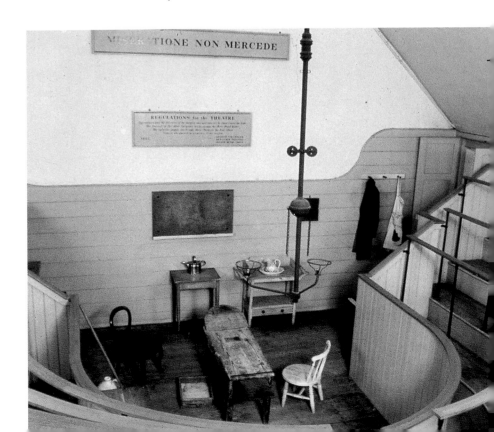

| 1400 | 1500 | 1600 | 1700 | 1800 | 1900 | 2000 |
|------|------|------|------|------|------|------|

B48 248 1210 ShS

**1493–1541**
Paracelsus
(Philippus Aureo
Theophrastus Bo
von Hohenheim)
Swiss doctor

**1543**
Vesalius A
(1514–64),
anatomist
publishes
about hur
based on
of bodies

**c.1510**
Ambr
surgeo
wound
pourir

Fleming
, Scottish
discovers

nall heart
aker invented

AT scan introduced
British engineer
odfrey Newbold
ounsfield
yhole surgery
st used

S recognized
disease

late
mi
Du

ROTHERHAM LIBRARY & INFORMATION SERVICES
This book must be returned by the date specified at the time of issue as the DATE DUE FOR RETURN.
The loan may be extended (personally, by post or telephone) for a further period if the book is not required by another reader, by quoting the above number / author / title.

LIS7a

**2000**
Scientists announce the
mapping of the human
es  genome

**2002**
An American company
announces it may have
an AIDS vaccine by 2005

that the heart pumps
blood around the body

**1865**
— Joseph Lister (1827–1912)
introduces antiseptics
— Queen Victoria uses
chloroform as an
anaesthetic

## Medicine and murder

There was a big medical school in Edinburgh, so the market for bodies to dissect was huge. So huge, in fact, that William Burke (1792–1829) and William Hare (c.1790–c.1860) found they couldn't meet the demand just by robbing graves. Burke owned a boarding house, and he and his companion took to murdering guests and selling their bodies. They murdered sixteen people and made a pretty penny before they were caught in 1829.

Nowadays people aren't so bothered about dissection, and many people actually leave their bodies to medical science to be studied after they die.

▶ **One of Burke and Hare's victims comes to a sticky end.**

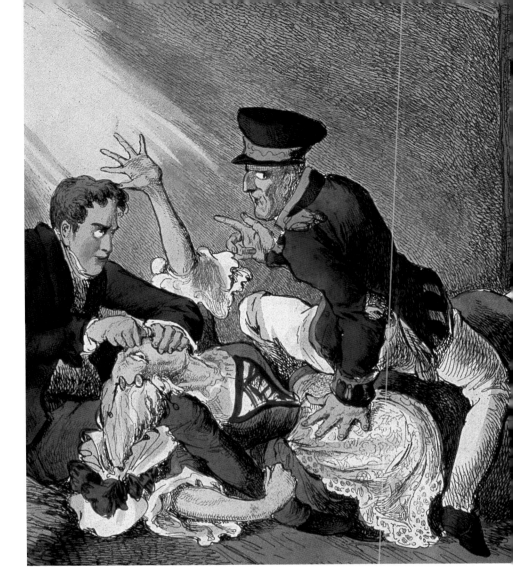

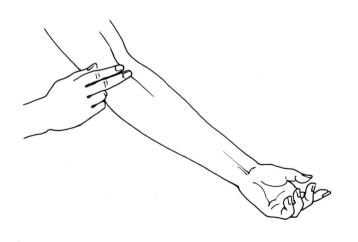

Here is an experiment to do at home. Hold out your right forearm and see if you can find a vein – they look like blue lines lying just under your skin. Now, run your finger along the vein from the crook of your elbow towards your wrist – but don't lift your finger off when you reach the end! You should find that the vein empties (the blueness disappears) and stays empty until you remove your finger. Now try it in the other direction, from your wrist to your elbow. You should find that the blood simply refills the vein as your finger moves. What direction do you think the blood is flowing in?

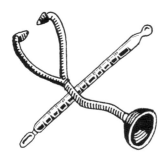

# Doctor doctor!
## *How did healers learn their trade?*

NOWADAYS doctors train for many years before they begin their work. But for as long as people have fallen ill there have been healers who have tried to make them better. Without written records it is hard to know what those healers would have been like in prehistoric times, but looking at societies which have kept their traditional ways of healing can give us some clues. In Australia, Aboriginal medicine men sing to their patients, or violently suck the infected part of the body. This is quite like rituals used by Native American healers, in which shamans call on supernatural powers to heal the sick. These rituals are used alongside simple herbal cures.

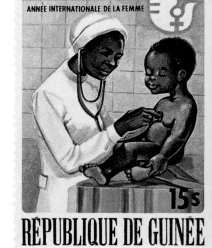

▲ Until quite recently most doctors were men. Now women all over the world train to be doctors.

### *Father to son*

Early civilizations also had doctors, although often they were not really separate from priests and magicians. In ancient Egypt all three worked together, each using a different approach. The priests called upon divine powers to heal the sick, magicians wove spells and incantations against evil spirits, and doctors examined their patients and prescribed remedies. There were no medical schools in ancient Egypt, and most doctors learned their trade from their families. Medical information was written on scrolls made from papyrus reed. These scrolls served as textbooks. They gave advice on how to examine the patient and what remedies to prescribe.

▼ A papyrus showing ancient Egyptian healing spells.

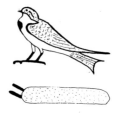

▲ These ancient Egyptian hieroglyphs spell out the word 'doctor' or 'physician'.

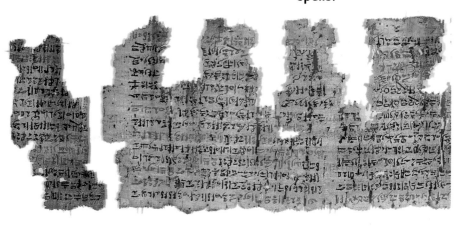

The tradition of healers training with their families was also found in ancient China, where sons studied with their fathers. Like Egyptian doctors, professional Chinese healers were expected to be familiar with a range of medical texts giving advice on symptoms and remedies. However, in both countries only the rich were able to afford professional doctors, and most people must have relied on friends, family and amateur healers for medical advice.

The same is true of classical Greece, where doctors were greatly respected. Medical schools flourished for the first time, although they were very different from those of today.

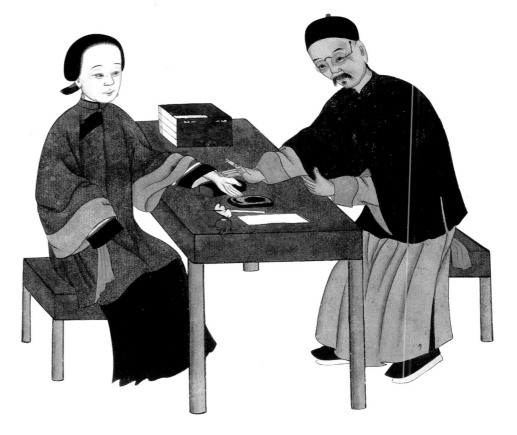

▲ An ancient Chinese doctor taking a pulse.

Greek physicians set up surgeries where they treated patients for a fee. The most famous medical school was on the island of Cos. Here the best-known doctor of all time, Hippocrates – the father of medicine – learned his trade. When he died his fame was so great people believed that the bees visiting the flowers on his grave made wax with special healing powers. Hippocrates had very specific ideas about doctors and their patients, which still form the basis of modern medicine today.

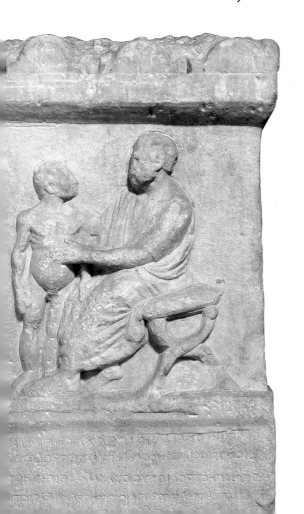

◄ A physician from the ancient Greek city of Athens at work in the early 2nd century AD.

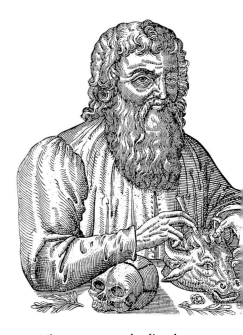

▲ Hippocrates, who lived in ancient Greece, was probably the most famous doctor of all time.

## The doctor's promise

Some of Hippocrates' ideas were gathered into the Hippocratic Oath – a series of promises which medical students had to make before they could begin their work. They promised to do everything in their power to help the sick, never to give a fatal poison to anyone, and never to tell anyone else about things they discussed in private with their patient.

At about the same time, doctors training in the Ayurvedic tradition in India had to make similar vows. The *Caraka Samhita*, a book written in AD 100, tells us that Ayurvedic doctors had to promise never to carry weapons, to speak the truth, to eat a vegetarian diet and to strive to bring relief to their patients. These ideals were sound enough, but unfortunately doctors in the ancient world didn't know enough about medicine to succeed every time their help was needed. So by the Roman era, people were quite doubtful about how useful doctors could be.

## Help for the rich – and the poor

There were no official examinations for doctors in ancient Greece or Rome. Students simply attached themselves to a teacher, and anyone could claim to be a doctor. For a long time in the Roman Empire almost all the doctors were immigrants from Greece, and many were slaves or ex-slaves. As time went by, the citizens of Rome became less afraid of the medical profession, and some doctors were even paid a fee by the civic authorities so that rich and poor alike could receive medical care. However, most doctors simply relied on their reputation to attract patients, and those who did well could make large amounts of money.

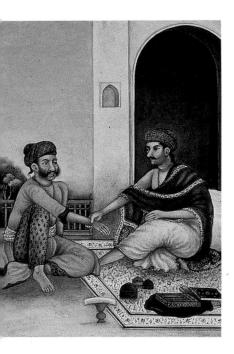

▲ A 19th-century Ayurvedic healer in India.

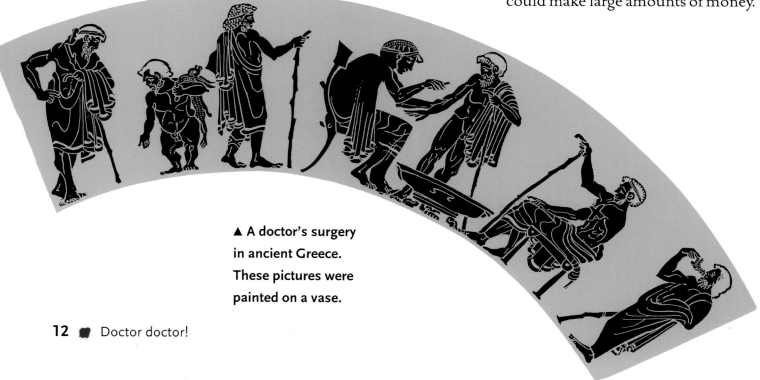

▲ A doctor's surgery in ancient Greece. These pictures were painted on a vase.

This was also the case in Europe right up until the Middle Ages. Most people couldn't afford to visit a doctor. By the thirteenth or fourteenth century AD, a whole range of healers offered cheaper alternatives. They included charmers, wise women, herbalists and piss prophets who claimed they could make a diagnosis by looking at a patient's urine. Some modern scientists have even suggested that these herbalists and wise women had a better understanding of natural remedies than medieval doctors, who relied on old-fashioned medical texts. Through trial and error, unqualified folk healers discovered a whole range of effective painkillers, digestive aids and soothing salves. Unfortunately, wise women were often confused with witches at this time and accused of doing harm rather than good.

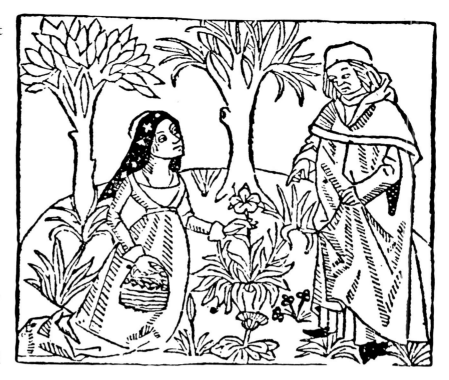

▲ Healers in the Middle Ages collecting herbs for their medicines.

▼ Medical students watching an operation in 1898.

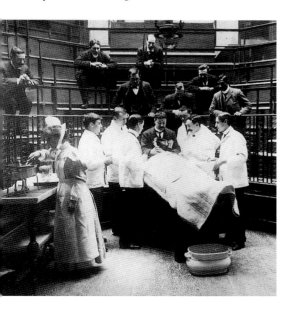

Over the last two hundred years, the governments of the world have gradually passed laws that have organized medicine and how it is practised. Doctors undergo long training programmes and have to pass many exams before they are allowed to treat patients. Most medicines are only available with a doctor's prescription, and most things modern doctors prescribe are unlikely to harm the patient. However, people still realise that going to see a doctor is not the only alternative if they fall ill, and today (as in medieval times) there are a whole range of therapists offering alternative advice on diet, exercise and herbal remedies.

▶ Nowadays medical students go through a rigorous training programme, with a lot of exams.

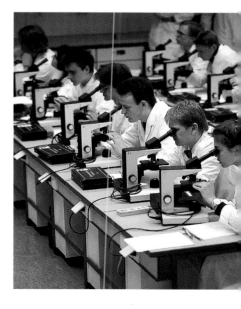

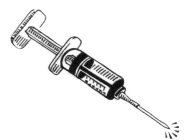

# Prevention is better than cure
## *Can healthcare and hygiene limit disease?*

Have you ever heard anyone say 'prevention is better than cure'? People have always tried to find ways of preventing illness, especially in the past, when they might not have trusted their doctors to make them better if they fell ill. There are all sorts of ways to limit the effects of disease, and some of them are quite simple.

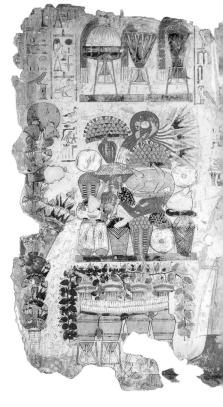

### *Clean clothes and healthy eating*

The hot climate in Egypt encourages harmful bacteria which spread disease. The ancient Egyptians did not know about bacteria, but because of the heat wore loose clothing. This allowed their skin to breathe and prevented a build-up of bacteria. They also washed their clothes often – unlike people hundreds of years later in medieval Europe, who were a pretty stinky bunch. Because the River Nile ran the length of Egypt it was easy to transport fresh fruit and vegetables from more fertile parts of the country to areas where they were harder to grow. Even poor

people in ancient Egypt ate a healthy, varied diet. Some ancient Egyptian houses have been found with wooden or stone seats with a removable bowl, which probably served as a kind of toilet. However, the typical Egyptian house, built of baked bricks and Nile mud, was infested by pests like rats and fleas that spread disease.

▲ This wall painting from the tomb of Nebamun shows an offering table piled with food. It shows what a varied, healthy diet the ancient Egyptians ate. On the table you can see wine jars, bread, meat, fruit and vegetables.

▶ Egyptian paintings show the comfortable, cool clothing worn by ancient Egyptians.

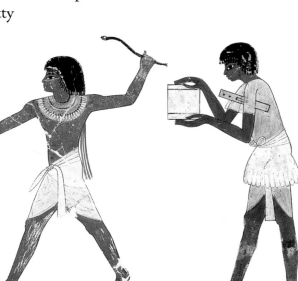

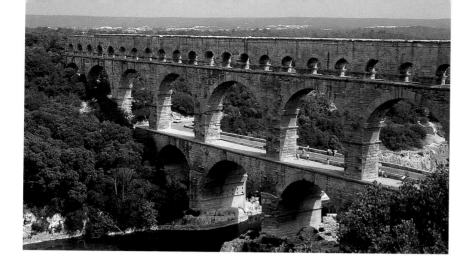

▲ The Pont du Gard, a Roman aqueduct that carried fresh water supplies into the city of Nemausus (modern Nîmes in France).

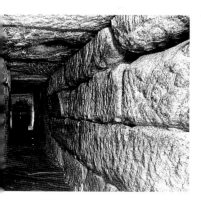

▼ A Roman sewer.

## Clean water

The ancient Romans, who liked to organize their towns and cities, were the first to think about improving public health. They built public toilets, sewers to carry away the waste material, and aqueducts to bring in fresh water supplies. The first aqueduct brought water into Rome in 312 BC. By AD 100 there were eight aqueducts carrying fresh water in tunnels and channels underneath the city streets. The water had to pass through settling tanks outside the city limits, so a lot of the harmful bacteria that cause diseases like dysentery would have been removed. Only the very wealthy could afford to have water piped directly into their houses, but a fresh water supply was only a short walk away for most Romans. Regular bathing also played an important part in Roman life. Most towns across the Roman Empire had at least one bath house, and entrance fees were cheap enough to allow even poorer Romans to make regular visits. The bath houses were places to get clean, to meet, to have a massage and even sometimes to have medical treatments.

Even in this organized world, life was not perfect. Despite their long, straight roads it was still difficult for the Romans to transport goods. It was hard to make sure that all the citizens of the Empire ate a varied diet, including fresh fruit and vegetables. Food shortages were common, and in bad times Rome's poor were issued with daily rations of corn to prevent them from starving. The sewer system in cities was a good idea, but there were times when the sewers overflowed, polluting rivers and spreading disease.

▼ This wall-painting shows a Roman party. Wealthy Romans ate a varied diet, but not all Romans were so lucky.

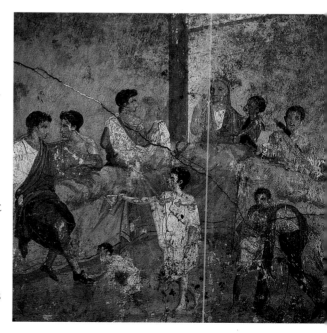

## Frightening illnesses

From the end of the fifth century AD the Roman Empire went into decline. Public health took a turn for the worse. In the medieval world, little was done to try to prevent disease, except in times of crisis. People were terrified of the rapid spread of diseases like the Black Death. In some cities, like Milan in Italy, victims were simply locked into their houses and left to die, for fear the plague should spread further. Leprosy was another disease that frightened medieval people, and lepers were forced to wear special clothing so that everyone would know they were infected. They also had to carry a handbell, which they rang to warn others they were approaching. Yet things were not completely bleak. The Christian Church played an important part in medieval life, and the Church believed that it was its Christian duty to care for the sick, who might spread infection if they were cared for in the community. Many monasteries set up hospitals where people who were ill could be cared for. Monks also cultivated herb gardens so they had all the necessary ingredients for their medicines close at hand.

## Overcrowding

Later on, from the 1700s onward, the Industrial Revolution led to a huge increase in the number of people living and working in cities. Living conditions were overcrowded, and children often had to work very long hours, just as their parents did. Many were poor and badly fed, and so they suffered from diseases like rickets and scurvy because they weren't getting enough vitamins and minerals from their diet. Dysentery and cholera – both of which are passed on by polluted water – were common, and people did not expect to live very long. Smallpox was also a huge problem, claiming hundreds of lives. One of the most important developments

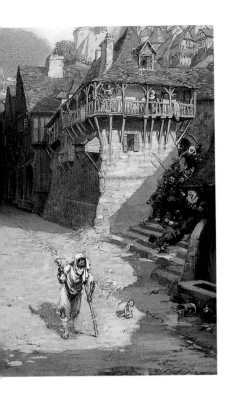

▲ People scramble to get away from a leper as they hear his bell.

# CHOLERA DISTRICTS.

### *LOOSENESS of the BOWELS is the Beginning of CHOLERA.*

Thousands of Lives may be saved by attending in Time to this Complaint, which should on no account be *neglected* by either Young or Old, in Places where the Disease prevails.

When CRAMPS IN THE LEGS, ARMS, or BELLY are felt, with LOOSENESS or SICKNESS AT STOMACH, when Medical Assistance is not at hand, *Three Tea-spoonsfull of* MUSTARD POWDER *in Half a Pint of warm Water*, or the same Quantity of warm Water with as much COMMON SALT as it will melt, should be taken as a Vomit; and after the Stomach has been cleared out with more warm Water, TWENTY-FIVE DROPS OF LAUDANUM should be taken in a small Glass of any agreeable Drink.

HEATED PLATES or PLATTERS to be applied to the BELLY and PIT of the STOMACH.

As Persons run considerable Risk of being infected by visiting those suffering from this Disease in crowded Rooms, it is most earnestly recommended that only such a Number of Persons as are sufficient to take care of the Sick be admitted into the Room.

*Central Board of Health,
Council Office, Whitehall,* 15th Feb. 1832.                    W. MACLEAN, *Secy.*

◀ These instructions were displayed in 1832 to try and minimize the harmful effects of cholera.

in public health was the discovery that a vaccination could be used to protect people from catching smallpox.

## Vaccination

Vaccination was the brainchild of an English doctor, Edward Jenner (1749–1823). He had noticed in his country surgery that farmers who suffered from cowpox (a much less serious disease) never caught smallpox afterwards. In 1796 Jenner carried out experiments on an eight-year-old boy. He deliberately infected the boy with contagious matter from a cowpox pustule. He later tried to infect the boy with smallpox and – luckily for both doctor and patient – his theory proved correct. Jenner was not the first doctor to try to use this method – but he was the first to have widespread success with vaccination. Nowadays vaccination programmes across the world have helped to control diseases like polio and typhus.

Over the years most countries have made all sorts of improvements in public health. Better sewage systems have been created, clean water supplies provided, hospitals built and most people – even in poorer countries – have access to some sort of medical care. It is hard for us to imagine what it must have been like to live at a time when death and disease were part and parcel of everyday life.

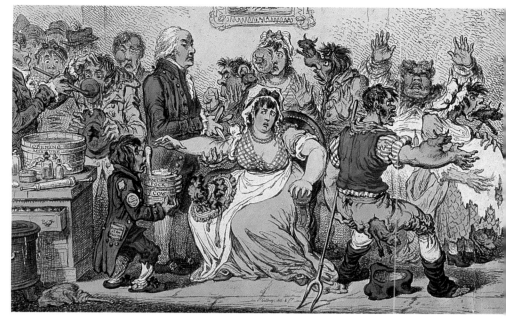

▲ This cartoon shows Edward Jenner, the inventor of the smallpox vaccination, with some of his patients.

▼ Postcards from the early 20th century promoting health care and hygiene.

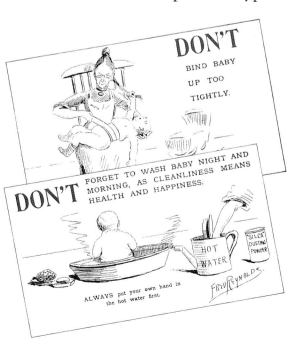

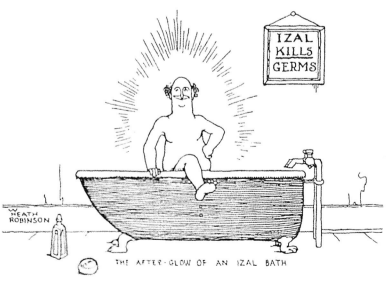

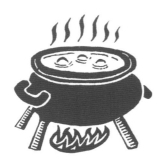

# Charms, spells and healing gods
## *Magic and religion in medicine*

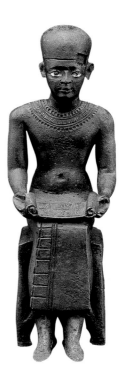

PREHISTORIC people didn't know the scientific reasons for illness, so they often blamed evil spirits or supernatural causes. This continued for a long time. Today, some people still carry lucky charms and say prayers for sick relatives.

### *Healing gods*

Belief in magical cures and healing gods has been around since prehistoric times. Cave paintings in France show human figures, who may have been doctor priests, wearing animal masks and performing ritual dances. We think these early sorcerers used a mixture of charms, amulets, spells and herbal medicines to heal the sick.

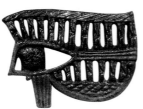

◄ Ancient Egyptians believed the Eye of Horus had special healing powers.

The civilizations of ancient Egypt, Greece and Rome each created their own magical and religious ways of healing. In ancient Egypt Horus and Imhotep were the gods of medicine. Like many ancient peoples the Egyptians believed that disease could be caused by demons and evil spirits, and the magical and medical papyri are full of spells and incantations for warding off evil and healing the sick.

Imhotep (*above*) was worshipped as a god of medicine in ancient Egypt. (*below*) Asklepios became a god of medicine in ancient Greece and Rome.

In ancient Greece Apollo was the god of healing. However, a cult also grew up around the doctor god Asklepios, the son of Apollo, and temples were built in his honour in Greek cities and towns. Patients slept in the temples in the hope that the god would send them a dream telling them how to cure their illness.

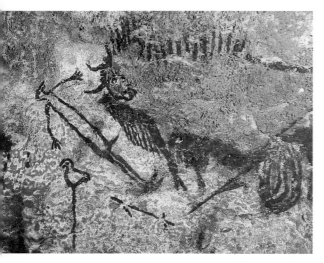

▲ The human figure in this prehistoric cave painting may have been a medicine man or shaman, about 15,000 years ago.

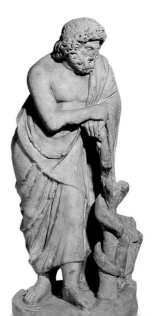

Later on, the Romans adopted Asklepios (calling him Aesculapius). Romans made sacrifices to Aesculapius and held festivals celebrating the god. One of the temple rituals involved the patient being visited by a snake. Does the symbol of the snake curled round a staff look familiar? It is still used by chemists today. Hoping to be cured, people also left clay, wood or stone models of the diseased parts of their bodies at the temples. Archaeologists have found large numbers of these models, including legs, arms, feet, eyes and ears.

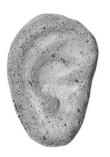

◄ This terracotta ear is one of the offerings left by Greek and Roman patients at healing shrines.

It is not so strange that people turned to magic and religion in a world where sickness and death were always around the corner, and ways of treating illness were often expensive and unreliable. In fact, people believed in evil spirits and magical cures all over the world. In Persia, Ahura Mazda, the god of light and good, was responsible for health and hygiene. In Arabia, jinn (evil spirits) were blamed for bringing sickness and death. The Chinese thought that sickness was brought by an evil wind and was cured by exorcising the evil spirits, or wearing charms and amulets.

## Punishments

In medieval Europe, the Church taught that illness and death were sent by God as punishments. Certain diseases such as leprosy were associated with sin. People made pilgrimages to the tombs of holy men and women where they left offerings of wax and metal models of parts of the human body. In some countries at this time people also thought that the king could help cure one disease simply by touching the sick person.

Miraculous cures, witchcraft and sorcery were used to heal the sick in Europe until just over a century ago. In many parts of the world, such as Africa and Asia, healers still include traditional charms among their remedies. In the West, people continue to blame divine powers for certain illnesses. Some people believe the disease AIDS is a punishment sent by God.

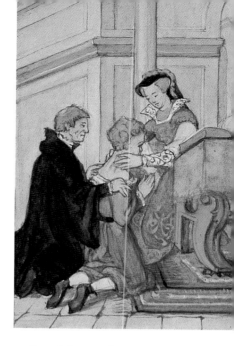

▲ Scrofula was known as the 'King's Disease'. People believed it could be cured by the touch of a royal person (this is Queen Mary I).

Suffering from a toothache? Why not try one of our medieval cures? Take a piece of paper and write out on it three times 'Jesus Christ, for mercy's sake, take away this toothache'. Now fold the paper up very tightly and throw it on the fire. (Be careful to make sure that there is an adult around to help you!) If everything goes according to plan, your toothache should go away . . .

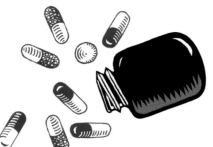

# Why take a pill for every ill?
## *Lotions, potions and herbal cures*

Today, hospitals and pharmacies are filled with all kinds of drugs, pills, lotions and creams. There is a treatment for most illnesses, and most are very easy to take. Modern drugs have been through a whole range of tests to make sure they don't have any harmful side effects. Although sometimes with very strong drugs – such as those used to treat cancer – people have to accept that they may feel worse before the treatment makes them better.

Most modern pharmacies also have a herbal section, where people can buy remedies made from plants and herbs. Some people prefer to use herbal remedies rather than chemical medicines because they believe herbal cures heal the body more naturally. But where did all these medicines come from? And how did people find out which plants and chemicals cured each disease?

### Mud and manure

People have been using medicines to cure disease for thousands of years. In fact, people in the past have used all kinds of weird and wonderful ingredients in their treatments. The ancient Egyptians used excrement to treat a whole range of diseases. They prescribed human excrement, and the excrement of crocodiles, pelicans and lizards. They also used mud from the River Nile, granite, bile collected from wild animals, and metals in their medicines. It must have been very difficult to collect some of the ingredients – such as tortoise bile or pelican poo!

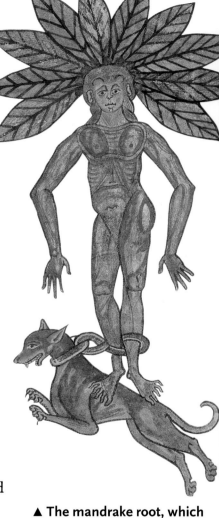

▲ The mandrake root, which resembles a human body, has been used in medicine since Roman times. In the Middle Ages dogs were used to pull up the root, because people believed that mandrakes would kill whoever uprooted them.

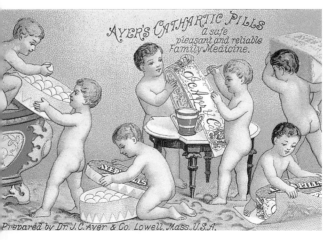

AYER'S CATHARTIC PILLS
a safe
pleasant and reliable
Family Medicine.

Prepared by Dr. J. C. Ayer & Co. Lowell, Mass. U.S.A.

◄ A 19th-century advertisement for a pill to cure all ills.

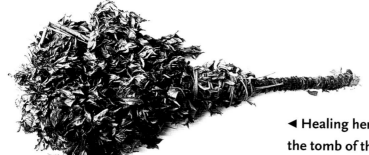

Pliny (AD 23–79), a famous Roman writer, collected together and listed a huge number of treatments. To cure a wild dog's bite he used badger, cuckoo and swallow excrement, and mouse excrement was prescribed to sweeten sour breath. It is hard to imagine people believing that these cures really worked, but until the eighteenth century doctors continued to prescribe remedies that included very strange ingredients, such as pearls, woodlice, unicorn's horn and frogspawn.

## The salt, the sweet and the sour

Some medicines people have taken in the past seem strange to us, but lots of old remedies were quite effective. Many are still used in some form by doctors today. The ancient Egyptians knew that opium, made from a type of poppy, was good for relieving pain. Opium is an ingredient of the modern drug morphine. Another remedy they used involved salt, which was rubbed on to cuts and sores and held in place with a bandage. Salt makes the cut sting, but

◀ Healing herbs found in the tomb of the Egyptian king Tutankhamun.

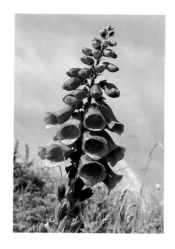

▲ Extracts from foxglove plants (digitalis) are still used to treat heart problems. But beware – foxglove plants are poisonous when growing!

▼ In China and Thailand medicine made from parts of the bodies of tigers are thought to have healing powers.

it has many healing properties. (Next time you get a mouth ulcer or a sore throat, try gargling with salt water. You may be surprised at how effective it is.)

The legendary Chinese Emperor Shen Nung, the 'father of Chinese medicine', who ruled China more than four and a half thousand years ago around 2737 BC, wrote a herbal manual that listed 365 herbs, poisons and remedies. Not all of the Emperor's treatments worked, but some are still used today. Good examples are kaolin, which is an excellent treatment for stopping diarrhoea, and rhubarb, which has the opposite effect.

Buddhist monks in India were only allowed a few belongings, but their monastic rule stated that they had to carry five simple medicines wherever they went, including fresh butter, honey and molasses. Early Indian herbal manuals teach about the healing properties of plants and, like the Chinese manuals, list hundreds of useful ingredients.

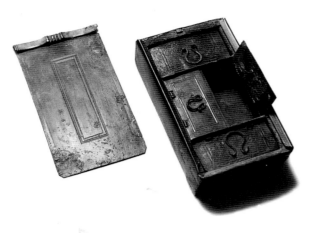

▲ In Roman times boxes like this one were used to hold medicines.

## Sugar and spice

The ancient Greeks also used herbal manuals, although they were quite cautious about prescribing remedies more complicated than honey and water, or honey and vinegar. The most famous Greek pharmacologist, Dioscorides (c. AD 40 – c. 90), wrote five books describing 600 medicinal plants. More adventurous Roman doctors travelled all over the Roman Empire learning about herbs and medicines from far-away places. Roman doctors knew that wine and vinegar could be used as antiseptics, and prescribed a range of soothing aloes and balsams. The sheer size of the Roman Empire meant that spices from far-off lands were available, at least to the wealthy.

## D.I.Y. medicine

Exotic ingredients continued to be popular until the Middle Ages. Medieval doctors used the recipes written down by Greek and Roman healers, and medieval apothecaries sold spices in their shops as well as medicines. Medieval healers also used a whole range of common-sense herbal cures, which had been passed down from generation to generation. These used free, locally-growing plants rather than expensive foreign ingredients. It is amazing how much has been discovered about the healing powers of plants simply through trial and error, and until recently this practical do-it-yourself medicine was still used by country people.

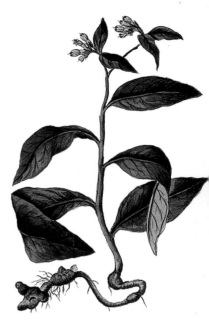

▲ Comfrey is a traditional cure for sprains and bruises as well as broken bones.

▼ A page from a 12th-century herbal giving information about herbs and their healing properties.

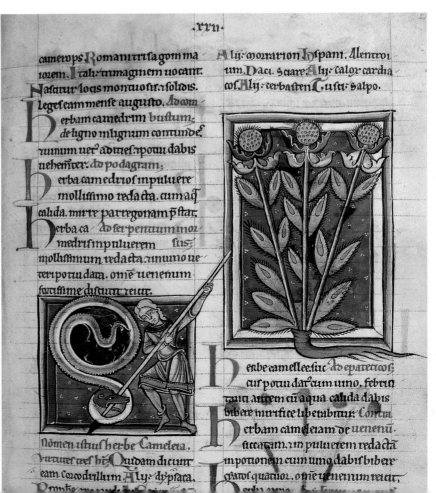

Older people may remember having nasty cuts bound in spiders' webs to make them heal without a scar, or having broken limbs healed with the herb comfrey (also known as knitbone). Many modern medicines are based on remedies that have been used for hundreds of years – like aspirin, which comes from the bark of the willow tree.

However, not all doctors continued to prescribe natural, herbal cures. During the early 16th century the Swiss doctor Paracelsus (1493–1541) flew in the face of tradition, and started to prescribe chemicals such as mercury, antimony, arsenic and sulphur. He is said to be the author of more than 600 works, although he claimed to scorn book learning and publicly burned the books of Galen and Hippocrates. He rejected many traditional medicines as old-fashioned, and encouraged the use of a whole range of new ingredients.

## A mouldy cure

Medicines continued to be improved, but it wasn't until the twentieth century that really spectacular developments took place. After the First World War (1914–18) a Scottish doctor called Alexander Fleming (1881–1955), worked on wounds and skin infections. He discovered penicillin, a mould which

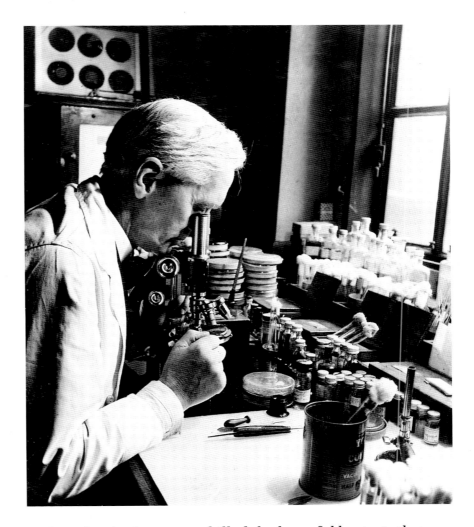

▲ Alexander Fleming at work in his laboratory.

▼ Penicillin, the world's first known antibiotic. In 1928 Alexander Fleming discovered that penicillin could kill harmful bacteria.

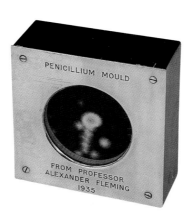

killed the harmful bacteria that caused blood poisoning. Penicillin, along with a range of other antibiotics, didn't seem to have any harmful side effects, and antibiotics are still used to treat many illnesses and infections. In recent years, all sorts of treatments have become available, and modern doctors use a mixture of herbal and chemical medicines to treat everything from depression to cancer. But we still cannot cure the common cold.

# The flash of the blade and the sound of the saw
## *Surgery through the ages*

As LONG as there have been doctors there have been surgeons too. Surgeons treat illness or disease by operating: cutting, drilling, splinting and stitching. An Indian book about medicine – the *Susruta Sanhita*, written more than 1600 years ago – tells us that surgery is the oldest of the medical arts, and archaeologists think people probably used surgery at least 7,000 years ago!

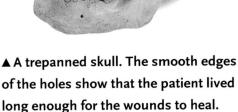

▲ A trepanned skull. The smooth edges of the holes show that the patient lived long enough for the wounds to heal.

### A hole in the head

One of the most ancient operations is known to doctors today as trepanning. In trepanning, a hole is cut or drilled into the skull to ease a build-up of pressure inside. Skulls with these kinds of marks have been found in France, Egypt, South America and the islands of the Pacific. Archaeologists can tell from the skulls they have found that some of the patients survived. It must have been a very painful operation, especially without an anaesthetic. Modern doctors use anaesthetics so that they can operate on patients without hurting them. A general anaesthetic makes the patient fall soundly asleep so they don't feel anything. A local anaesthetic stops the patient from feeling pain in a particular part of the body.

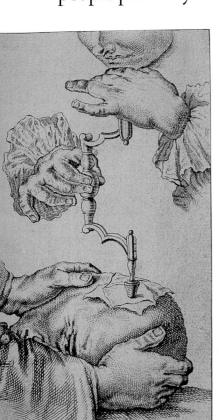

▲ This poor fellow is being trepanned.

### Early surgeons at work

But what else could surgeons in the ancient world do? We know quite a lot about this because some of these healers wrote books describing their work. One of the oldest of these books comes from Egypt. It is written on papyrus and is more than 3,500 years old.

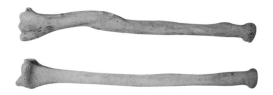

▲ Arm bones from ancient Egypt. One has been broken and healed slightly crooked.

Magical and medical papyri tell us that Egyptian doctors were able to set broken bones in ox bone splints, wrapped in bandages soaked in resin – rather like having your leg put in plaster today. Looking at Egyptian mummies shows how well some of their fractures healed. The Egyptians also knew how to dress wounds and treat abscesses.

Archaeologists haven't been able to find any recognizable surgical instruments from ancient Egypt, but they have found many from the Roman Empire. The Romans were skilled at making surgical instruments out of metals such as copper, bronze, iron and brass. As well as being able to set bones and treat abscesses, the Roman healers tackled a wide range of operations, from the amputation of arms and legs to the removal of in-growing eyelashes. Some were skilled eye surgeons.

## New noses

As a general rule, that was as complicated as surgery got in the ancient world – with one strange exception. In India the punishment for one offence was for the guilty person's nose to be cut off. As a result Indian doctors came up with a way of rebuilding the nose using skin cut from the cheek and reed tubes to keep the nostrils open. This is one of the earliest known forms of plastic surgery!

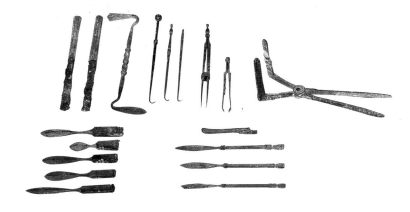

▲ These ancient Roman surgical instruments look surprisingly like modern surgical tools.

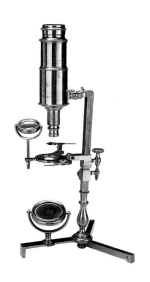

▲ An 18th-century microscope. The invention of the microscope in the 16th century enabled doctors to study micro-organisms for the first time.

▶ Surgery in the 12th century could be a nasty business.

## Pain and danger

As medicine became more advanced surgery started to improve. However, surgery was a painful and dangerous business in a world without anaesthetics and without any proper antiseptics. You probably know that if you get a cut, you need to clean it and put antiseptic cream on it to stop it from becoming infected. However, doctors didn't find out about the tiny organisms that cause blood poisoning and other infections until after the microscope was invented by Dutch spectacle-makers in the late sixteenth century.

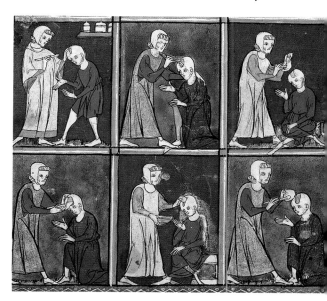

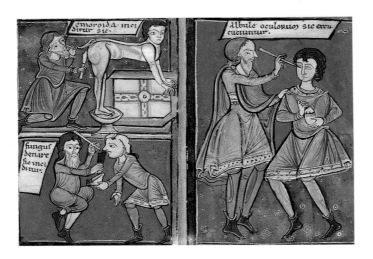

◀ Surgery in the 14th century.

▶ **Medieval surgeons mistakenly believed that bleeding their patients would help them to get better.**

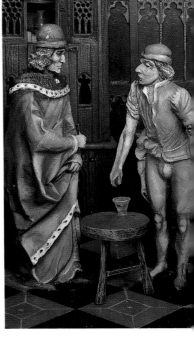

Imagine what it must have been like to have a limb amputated in the past… strong assistants had to hold down the poor patient. The skin was cut with a knife and the bone with a saw. In early amputations, the wound was cauterized with hot oil to stop the bleeding. This continued to be the case until 1536, when a French army surgeon called Ambrose Paré (c.1510–90) perfected a system for tying off the ends of veins and arteries.

Without anaesthetics, the shock of the pain could have killed the patient if infection didn't. Because of this, speed was extremely important, and doctors prided themselves on how quickly they could carry out operations. One very famous doctor, Robert Liston (1794–1847), worked in London in the early 1800s. He could amputate a leg in less than two minutes. After cutting the skin he would place the knife between his teeth so he could speedily take up his

saw. But Robert Liston operated wearing dirty, bloody clothes, in a crowded operating theatre filled with foul-smelling odours and the screams of the patient. Surgery could only advance after two important discoveries were made.

▼ **Amputating a limb in the 16th century.**

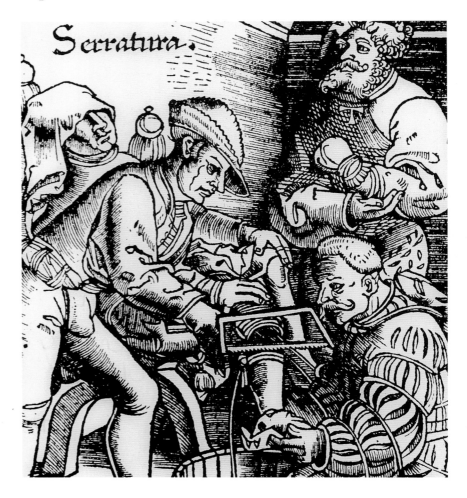

Serratura.

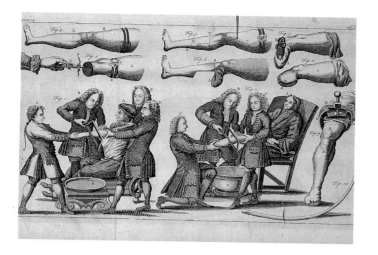

◄ These diagrams were drawn in the 18th century to show the best way to amputate arms and legs.

## Anaesthetics arrive . . .

The first discovery was that certain substances could be used to make patients drowsy. Doctors had experimented with hypnotism, but often had to resort to giving the patient large amounts of alcohol, so they would wake up with a hangover on top of everything else! Crawford Long (1815–78), an American doctor, first used a chemical called ether to put patients to sleep in 1842. Later, Queen Victoria made use of a similar substance – chloroform – during the birth of one of her children. These early anaesthetics were not perfect, but they still marked a vast improvement.

## . . . and antiseptics

Then in 1865 a Scottish doctor, Joseph Lister (1827–1912), made another important discovery. He introduced the use of antiseptic carbolic acid to clean surgical instruments and dress wounds. He even sprayed a fine carbolic mist in the operating theatre, which greatly reduced the risk of infection. Many more patients survived the operating theatre after these discoveries were made. Today surgeons wear clean clothing, face masks and throw-away gloves. Conditions have improved so much in modern operating theatres that highly skilled surgeons can do anything from removing in-growing toenails to replacing the human heart.

▲ Dr Lister and his assistants.

▼ A 21st century operating theatre.

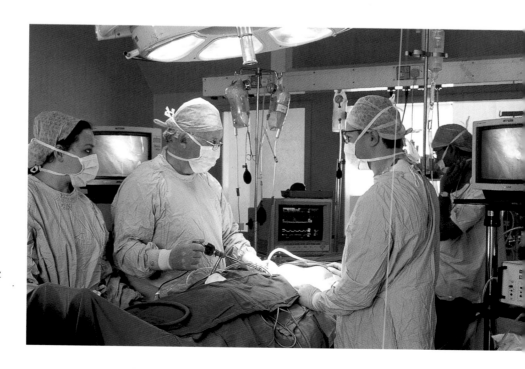

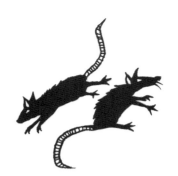

# Deadly diseases
## *Catch them if you can!*

MANY DISEASES were unknown to prehistoric people. In early times people found their food by hunting wild animals and gathering plants and nuts. Later, when people began to domesticate animals, they came into contact with all sorts of illnesses. Cows brought cowpox, which later became smallpox in human beings. Pigs and ducks gave us influenza, and horses brought the viruses that cause the common cold. Water polluted with animal wastes spread diseases like diphtheria, cholera and whooping cough. Towns and cities provided the perfect environment for rats, fleas and other pests that spread disease.

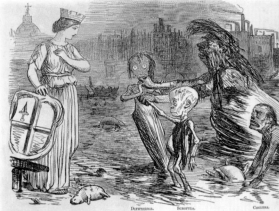

▲ A cartoon from the magazine Punch from 1858. The River Thames in London once carried all sorts of diseases in its polluted waters.

The people of the ancient Near East were the first to domesticate animals, and ancient Egyptian tomb paintings show that cattle were farmed in Egypt more than 5,000 years ago. Studying Egyptian mummies tells us that tuberculosis was already around in ancient Egyptian times. People caught tuberculosis from drinking infected cows' milk or eating infected meat. Some kinds of tuberculosis can damage the spine, so it's easy to tell whether an Egyptian mummy had the disease. Unfortunately, many other diseases kill without leaving any traces on the bones. So we can only find out about these illnesses when people in the past wrote about them.

▼ This painting from an Egyptian tomb shows ancient Egyptian farmers counting their herd of cattle.

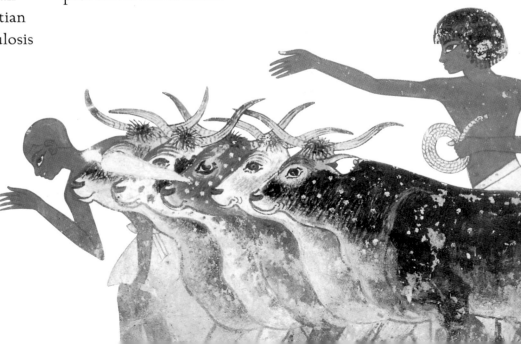

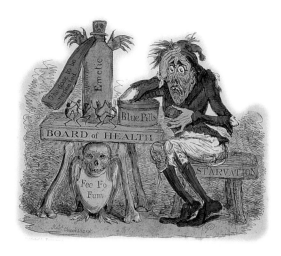

▲ Trying anything to cure cholera.

## Epidemics

We know that epidemics of diseases have occurred throughout history. A Greek historian records a plague – perhaps measles or smallpox – that killed a quarter of the Athenian army in 430 BC. The Romans also suffered from epidemics, and travellers could spread diseases far and wide across the huge Roman Empire. An unknown disease struck Rome in AD 165. The Roman army had been fighting in Mesopotamia (modern Iraq), and when the troops returned home they brought the sickness with them. The epidemic lasted fifteen years and stretched all the way from Gaul to Persia, killing many thousands of Roman citizens.

## Plague!

Then in AD 542 an even bigger epidemic broke out. It was probably bubonic plague – a disease carried by the fleas that live on rats. Roman doctors did not know much about the disease and so they had no effective way to treat it. Even the Roman Emperor Justinian (c. AD 482–565) became ill, although luckily for him he survived. The plague killed Roman officials and slaves alike. Hundreds of thousands died, and the epidemic may have been one of the things that contributed to the decline of the Roman Empire.

Bubonic plague struck again in the fourteenth century, when it was known as the Black Death. It was probably brought to Europe by Italian merchants returning from the Black Sea. Italian cities saw the first cases of the plague in 1347, and from Italy it spread across France, Germany, Holland and England, killing more than a quarter of the population. Doctors at the time did not know that the disease was spread by micro-organisms. They thought the infection was caused by the wrath of God and carried in foul-smelling mists called miasmas. Doctors wore protective leather aprons and strange beak-like masks filled with sweet-smelling herbs, and they burned incense in the bedrooms of the sick in an attempt to drive out the disease.

▶ A 14th-century plague doctor in special protective clothing.

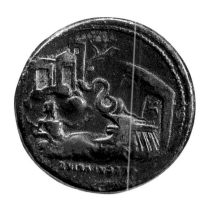

▲ A medallion showing Aesculapius coming to the rescue of Roman plague victims in 295 BC.

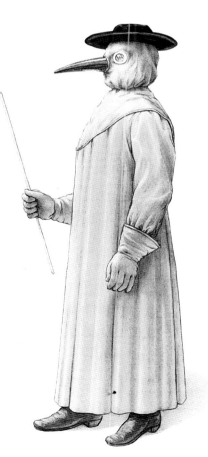

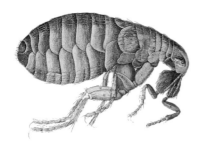

▲ We know now that fleas like this one carried plague.

Across Europe, cities struck by plague closed their gates to travellers. Orders were issued for all cats and dogs to be killed. But nothing the authorities did seemed to halt the spread of the plague. Terrified people looked for someone to blame, and Jews were accused of poisoning wells and deliberately spreading the plague. Many Jews were tortured or burned alive before Pope Clement VI declared that the Jews were innocent.

The Black Death ended in 1351, but in Europe bubonic plague continued to be a problem for hundreds of years. Officials did everything they could to limit the spread of plague. In many cities the sick were simply locked up in their houses and left to die. Huge pits were dug beyond the city limits to bury the bodies of the dead. Searchers were employed to go about and identify the houses where plague victims lived. Some families deliberately locked themselves in their homes, while others fled the cities. Those who remained took precautions not to come into contact with others, even paying for their food with money left in bowls of vinegar. Then the plague began to die out

in Europe. Perhaps people became immune to the disease, or perhaps the rats who carried the fleas did. No one is quite sure why, but the plague left England, Italy, France and Russia in the eighteenth century. The last great European plague epidemic was in Marseilles, France, in 1720, and the last epidemic in Asia and the United States was in the 1890s.

*Flu and measles*

Today you would be very surprised if a doctor said you were suffering from the plague. A more recent epidemic was a disease you probably associate with nasty winter weather and sore throats. It was an influenza epidemic,

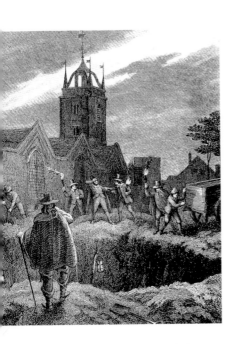

▲ During times of plague, city dwellers buried their dead in huge pits outside the city limits.

▶ Coughs and sneezes really do spread diseases! This government poster is urging cold sufferers to be careful not to spread their germs to other people.

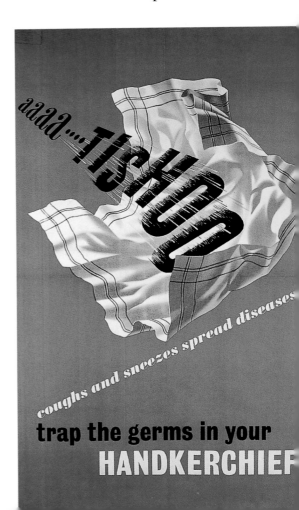

aaaa...TISHOO

coughs and sneezes spread diseases

trap the germs in your HANDKERCHIEF

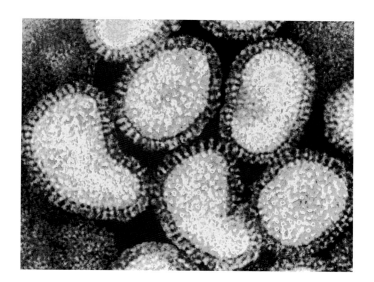

◄ An influenza virus seen through a microscope.

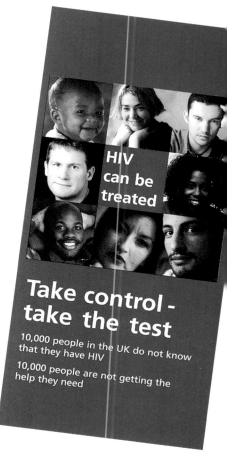

HIV can be treated

**Take control - take the test**

10,000 people in the UK do not know that they have HIV

10,000 people are not getting the help they need

▲ New diseases, like AIDS, are developing all the time. We may have to deal with many more diseases in the future.

which swept the world in 1918. It spread from Sierra Leone to the United States and Europe. Spanish flu, as it was called, killed 25 million people in six months – the deadliest epidemic since the Black Death. Sometimes seemingly harmless diseases can have devastating effects when people come into contact with them for the first time. The first Europeans to sail down the River Amazon in 1542 were almost immune to the effects of measles, but Amazonian Indians died in their hundreds when exposed to the disease.

But don't worry if you catch measles or flu. It's unlikely they will kill you off. In fact, since the Great Influenza Epidemic, there haven't been any disease disasters of this type. Living conditions across the world have improved, so people have better immune systems to fight disease. And immunization and treatment programmes have brought diseases like polio and tuberculosis under

control. However, new diseases such as HIV, the virus that causes AIDS, can still cause fear and suffering. When the disease was first identified in the 1980s there was a great panic, and some frightened people claimed that the sickness was a punishment from God. Does that sound familiar?

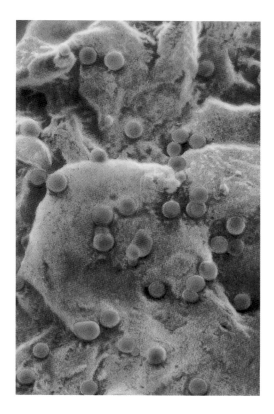

◄ A cell infected with the HIV virus. This virus causes the disease AIDS.

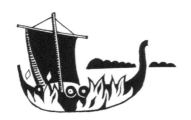

# Endings or beginnings?
## *Ways of dealing with death*

IN THE MODERN WORLD preventative medicine, better living conditions and improved medical treatments enable most people to live long lives. But until the twentieth century people didn't expect to live nearly as long. If you had lived over a hundred years ago, it is more than likely that by the age you are now, you would have lost some of your friends and family. This is still the case in many developing countries today.

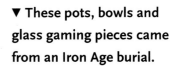

▲ This Iron Age warrior from Deal in eastern England was buried wearing his crown.

All over the world, from the last Ice Age – about 15,000 years ago – to the present day, people have developed ways of dealing with death. This is partly for practical reasons. Decomposing bodies are very smelly and can spread disease so, unless your community is on the move, dead bodies have to be disposed of by means such as burial or burning. Other rituals may have grown up to help the living with the grieving process. Losing somebody you love is very distressing. When it happens, having a set of rules and regulations to follow helps to draw people together in their time of need. It may also help grieving friends and relatives to believe that death is not the absolute end of that person's existence. The funeral ceremonies and burial practices of people in ancient Egypt, ancient Greece, Anglo-Saxon England, Viking Europe, and early America may be quite different from one another, but most of them have something in common – they show belief in the continuation of life after death.

### Graves and grave goods

As far back as Neolithic times – from around 5,000 BC – people were burying their dead in marked

▼ These pots, bowls and glass gaming pieces came from an Iron Age burial.

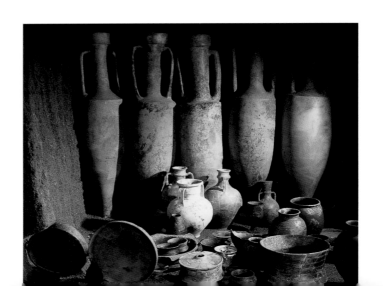

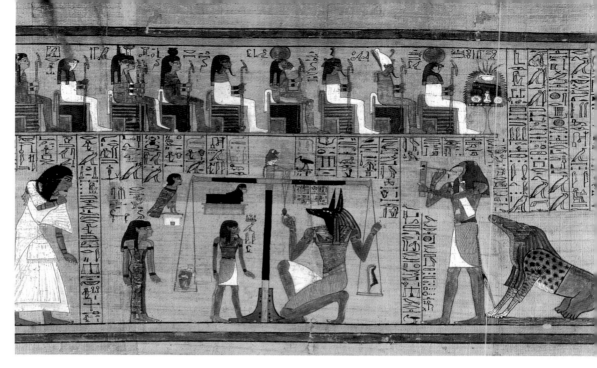

▶ A dead person faces the judgement of the gods in the ancient Egyptian 'weighing of the heart' ceremony.

▼ The ancient Egyptians mummified animals as well as people. Cats like this one were sacred to the goddess Bastet.

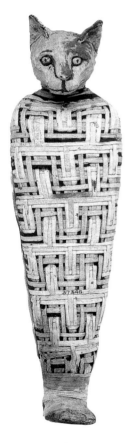

▶ Don't lose your head! This protective mummy-mask belonged to an ancient Egyptian priest.

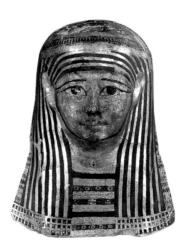

graves, with food, weapons and other useful items the dead person could take with them to the afterlife. We know this because archaeologists have discovered many Neolithic graves and investigated their contents. But the grave goods found in Neolithic burials are not nearly as spectacular as those found in the tombs of the ancient Egyptians. Egyptian graves even contained instructions on how to deal with the afterlife, written down in *The Book of the Dead*,

▶ This amulet is a heart scarab in the shape of the sacred scarab beetle. Scarab amulets were placed in the wrappings of Egyptian mummies as a protection.

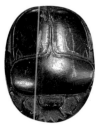

which included information on how to avoid injuries such as being bitten by a snake or dying for a second time. The ancient Egyptians believed it was important for the body of a dead person to reach the afterlife intact. They developed mummification so that the body could be preserved and placed in the tomb wrapped in bandages and encased in a protective coffin. One of the worst things that could happen to an Egyptian person in the afterlife was losing his or her head, so many mummies wore protective masks as well.

## Ferry across the River Styx

The ancient Egyptians were not the only ones to believe in an afterlife. The ancient Greeks thought that a dead person had to travel to an underworld ruled by the god Hades and guarded by the three-headed dog, Cerberus. To reach the underworld, the dead person had to cross over the River Styx, paying a fee to Charon the ferryman. Another river flowing through the underworld was the River Lethe. The Greeks believed that by drinking from the waters of Lethe, the river of forgetfulness, people lost the memory of everything that had happened to them before they died.

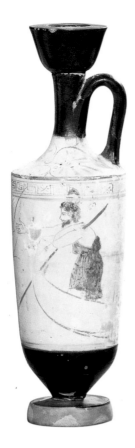

▲ This ancient Greek pot shows Charon, the ferryman who took the dead across the river Styx to the underworld.

## Ship burials

Ships and boats feature in the funerary rituals of other cultures too. One famous ship burial is at Sutton Hoo in eastern England. An Anglo Saxon king – perhaps the sixth-century king Raedwald – was laid in a great sea-going ship and a huge mound of earth was raised over it, burying the ship completely. It was not uncovered until 1939.

▼ A Viking sword found buried in a warrior's grave.

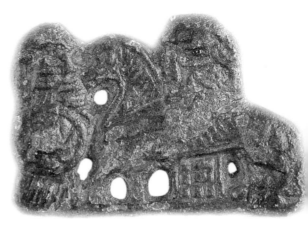

▲ A Viking warrior being welcomed into Valhalla.

In the Viking world it was important for warriors to fight bravely and honourably to make sure they would be allowed to enter the great hall of Valhalla when they died. Valhalla was the Viking paradise. Here warriors who had died on the battlefield feasted from dawn to dusk every day, completely healed of their wounds. The bodies of important kings or warriors were sometimes buried inside a longboat or Viking ship, with farming tools, kitchen utensils, food and drink.

## Funeral pyres

The Vikings and other peoples also disposed of dead warriors and kings by building a funeral bonfire, called a pyre, and burning the body.

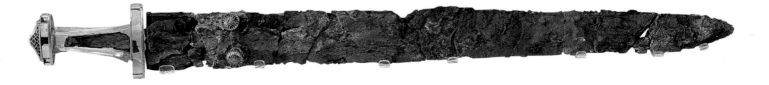

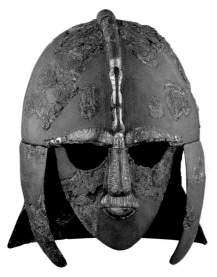

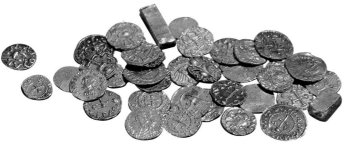

◄ The helmet and coins were among the grave goods discovered in a 6th-century ship burial at Sutton Hoo.

In some cases the dead man's widow was expected to throw herself on to the burning pyre to join her husband in death. This ritual was also once part of the Hindu way of life in India. There, widowhood was shameful and some women preferred to die rather than face life without a husband. Widows did not have to commit suicide to join their husbands in death, but it was considered very brave and praiseworthy to do so. Sometimes the widow would come to the funeral wearing full bridal make-up and clothes, as if she were going to marry her husband again. This practice was known in India as suttee or sati,

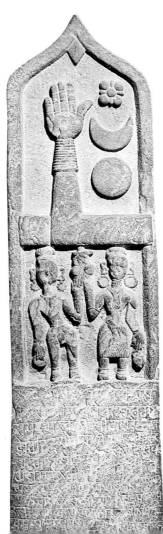

◄ This memorial stone commemorates a widow who committed sati in the 18th century. The upturned hand was a symbol often found on sati stones.

and it was banned in 1829. However, the last person to commit sati in India did so in 1987.

Sati was banned partly because the widows were taking their own lives. Suicide is frowned upon by most religions, and this plays an important part in modern arguments about euthanasia, or assisted death. Some people now argue that we are living too long, and that modern medicine can prolong life past the point where it is enjoyable. Euthanasia gives patients the right to request that their life be ended should their health worsen. This could mean turning off a life-support machine, or giving a lethal dose of pain-killing drugs. A large number of people are in favour of euthanasia, but many others are not. Euthanasia is still illegal everywhere except Japan, Columbia, the Netherlands and the state of Oregon in the United States. Many doctors feel that it goes against their principles of only using their knowledge to help the sick.

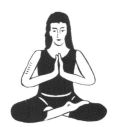

# What's the alternative?
## *Complementary medicine in the Western world*

A<small>N 'ALTERNATIVE'</small> therapy is one that uses healing techniques different from those of conventional doctors. Alternative therapies have gained in popularity in recent years, but they are not an entirely new development. People have been complaining for a long time that conventional medicine is blinkered and doesn't take into account all the treatments available. In fact, some people believe that conventional Western medicine is sick itself, because it relies on chemicals and bold surgical methods rather than natural cures.

### A kick-start cure

One of the first alternative therapies to become really popular was homeopathy. It was invented in the early 1800s. Homeopathy works on the theory that one disease drives out another. The body of a sick person shows symptoms of the illness. Homeopathic treatments give the sick person a controlled amount of something that causes symptoms similar to the illness. This starts up the body's own healing ability. So somebody with insomnia (inability to sleep) and trembling might be prescribed a very small dose of coffee. Coffee stimulates the body and drinking strong coffee at night can stop people sleeping. So in theory a small dose of coffee should trigger the body's natural defences and kick-start the healing process.

### Straight spines

Osteopathy and chiropractic are therapies that grew up in the later 1800s. Both osteopaths and chiropractors concentrate on the spine, manipulating the bones and joints and popping bones that are out of line back into place.

▼ An osteopath treating a patient.

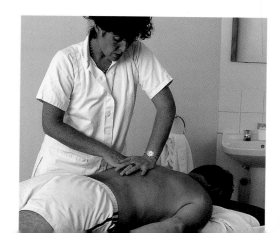

▲ A 19th-century plan for a homeopathic medical college in New York City.

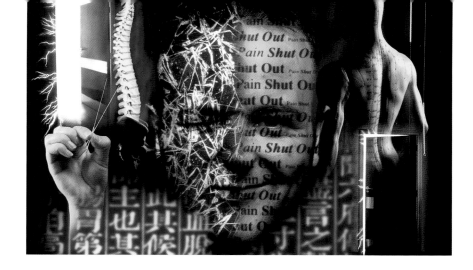

◀ Acupuncture treatment has become popular with people all around the world.

Today there are almost as many alternative therapists as there are conventional doctors. Many doctors actually refer some of their patients to an alternative therapist for treatment. Alternative therapies are popular in countries such as Britain, France, the United States and Canada, where one in five people uses meditation, massage acupuncture, hypnosis or other treatments. Recently the British Medical Association recommended that acupuncture should be made freely available on the National Health Service. In hospital wards which look after people who are dying, it is not unusual to find nurses using aromatherapy or reflexology to ease their patients' suffering. Slowly but surely, conventional Western medicine is opening its eyes to the wide range of therapies that can help the sick.

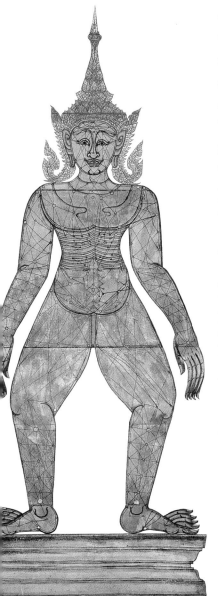

▼ A diagram of pressure points and energy flows in the human body, from a Thai manuscript.

## Chinese needles

One of the most popular alternative therapies today is acupuncture. This is a technique originally developed by the Chinese some 5,000 years ago. It works on the principle that energy flows through channels in the body and using special pressure points can affect the flow of energy. The acupuncturist puts very fine needles into the pressure points that relate to particular illnesses or parts of the body to unblock the energy flow and heal the patient.

## Toe hold

Reflexology also uses pressure points, but in reflexology the points are all on the foot. The reflexologist finds out what the patient's symptoms are and massages the feet in the relevant place. Next time you get a headache, try massaging your big toes all around the edges and on the sole. You might find it as helpful as taking an aspirin.

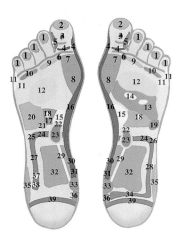

▲ This diagram shows the reflexology pressure points on the soles of the feet.

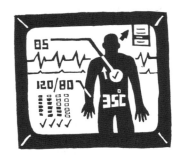

# What now and whatever next?
## *The future of medicine*

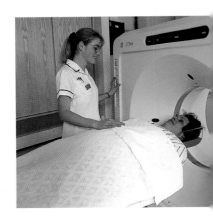

▲ A patient entering a CAT scanner.

Duracking the last hundred years medicine has made huge advances. Surgery was once difficult and dangerous, but now doctors can remove and replace organs – even the heart – in safe, antiseptic operating theatres. The new heart can then be checked and controlled with an artificial device called a pacemaker. Tiny babies, born weeks early, can be kept alive in special incubators until they are big enough to survive on their own. And in Intensive Care units, people whose hearts and lungs have stopped working can be hooked up to machines that will pump blood and breathe for them.

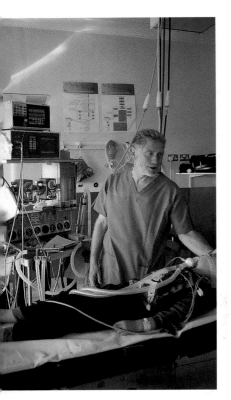

▲ An anaesthetist looking after a patient in a modern operating theatre.

X-rays and CAT scans allow doctors to see detailed pictures of the inside of the human body without having to cut patients open. In fact, it's thanks to CAT scans and X-rays that palaeopathologists know so much about the insides of ancient mummies. And scientists can make artificial replacements for parts of the body that go wrong, such as hip joints and heart valves.

## Looking forward

What does the future hold? One of the important things to remember is that most of these exciting developments are only happening in wealthy countries. Many people in the developing world still suffer from inadequate health care, so one thing we could hope for is that better medical care will be available to everyone.

In the developed world doctors can carry out some operations through a very small hole in the body. This is called keyhole surgery and the surgeon uses tiny cameras, lasers and robots. Doctors hope to carry out many more operations this way.

As medicine becomes more advanced, people are living longer. Doctors are having to deal with more of the diseases that come with old age. These include rheumatism and arthritis (diseases that make the joints sore and swollen) and Alzheimer's disease (which can make people forgetful and confused).

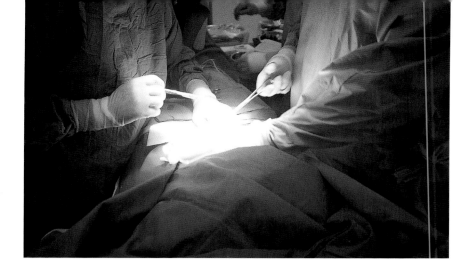

## New diseases

New diseases, such as AIDS, are developing all the time. And there is still no cure for many older diseases such as multiple sclerosis and some forms of cancer. So scientists are searching for new remedies. One of the places they are looking for help is in our genes – the complex pattern books inside our bodies that decide what we look like and what inherited diseases we may have. Scientists are currently experimenting on copying and altering genes.

▼ Is this how surgery might look in the future?

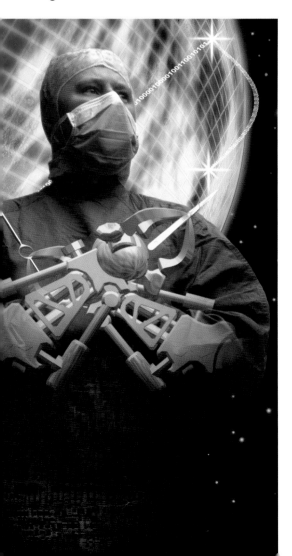

Dolly the sheep was the first ever cloned animal. Some genetically modified crops can resist plant diseases.

However, genetic engineering has been criticized for taking medicine too far. There are many questions for modern medicine. Should doctors try to prolong life indefinitely? Should they be allowed to tamper with our genetic make-up? Or might this start off a chain of unpredictable and perhaps dangerous events?

What do you think?

▲ Surgery has come a long way in the last 200 years, and new surgical techniques are developing all the time.

▼ A sweater made from the wool of Dolly, the first genetically engineered sheep. In the early 1990s it would have been impossible to clone a sheep. What will the next ten years bring?

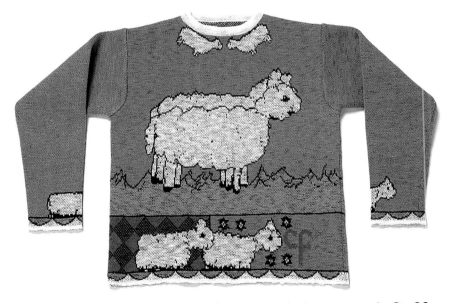

# Index

# Further reading

## For children

*A Doctor's Life – A Visual History of Doctors and Nurses Through the Ages*, by Rod Storring (Heinemann, 1998)
*How Your Body Works*, by Judy Hindley & Colin King (Usborne, 2003)
*The Human Body*, edited by Dr Tony Smith (Dorling Kindersley, 2002)
*Incredible Body* by Stephen Biestly (Dorling Kindersley, 1998)
*Medicine and Health through Time: an SHP Development Study*, by Ian Dawson & Steve Coulson (John Murray, 1996)
*Understanding Your Muscles and Bones* (Usborne, 2003)
*Understanding Your Body* (Usborne, 2003)

## For adults

*Ancient Egyptian Medicine*, by John F. Nunn, (British Museum Press, 1996)
*Doctors and Diseases in the Roman Empire*, by Ralph Jackson (British Museum Press, 1988)
*History of Medicine*, by Roberto Margotta (Hamlyn, 1996)
*Medicine and Society in later Medieval England*, by Carole Rawcliffe (Sutton, 1995)
*Medicine's 10 Greatest Discoveries*, by Mayer Friedman & Gerald W. Friedland (Yale University Press, 2000)
*Of Greatest Benefit to Mankind: A Medical History of Humanity from Antiquity to the Present*, by Roy Porter (HarperCollins, 1997)
*Wisdom, Memory and Healing* by Gabrielle Hatfield (Sutton, 1999)

# Timeline

c. stands for 'circa', the Latin word for 'around'

| 1 ¾ million years ago | 5000 BC | 1000 BC | 500 BC | AD 1 | AD 500 | AD 1000 | 1300 |
|---|---|---|---|---|---|---|---|

**1 ¾ million years ago – 10,000 years ago:**
Pleistocene Epoch. Last Ice Age

**c. 8000 – 4000**
Neolithic (New Stone Age) people begin to farm for the first time and live in villages

**c. 3100 – 332**
Rule of the pharaohs in Egypt

**4th – 5th centuries BC**
Classical Greece

**753**
City of Rome founded

**c. 460 – c. 375**
Hippocrates of Cos, Greek doctor

**c. 800**
Start of the Iron Age in Europe

**c. 221 BC – AD 1911**
Imperial China

**23 – 79**
Pliny (Gaius Plinius Secundus) Roman writer

**c. 40 – c. 90**
Pedanius Dioscorides, Greek doctor and writer

**129 – c. 216**
Galen of Pergamum, Greek doctor and writer

**476**
Last emperor of the Western Roman Empire overthrown

**c. 482 – 565**
Justinian, Emperor of the Eastern Roman Empire

**542**
Plague epidemic in Roman Empire

**c. 5th – 15th centuries AD**
The Middle Ages in Europe

**1342 – 1352**
Reign of Pope Clement VI

WITHDRAWN

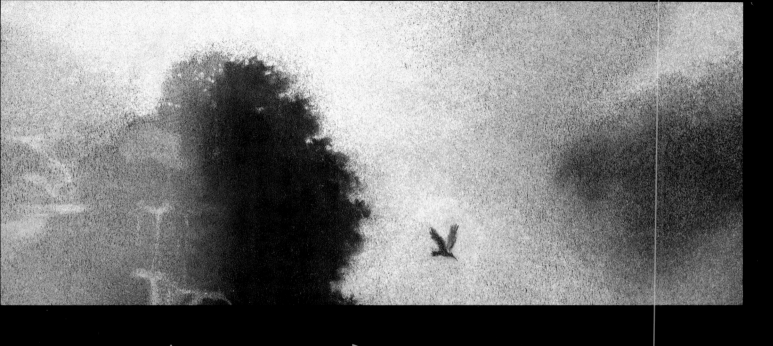

# African Beginnings

# AFRICAN BEGINNINGS

JAMES HASKINS & KATHLEEN BENSON

PAINTINGS BY FLOYD COOPER

LOTHROP, LEE & SHEPARD BOOKS · MORROW

NEW YORK

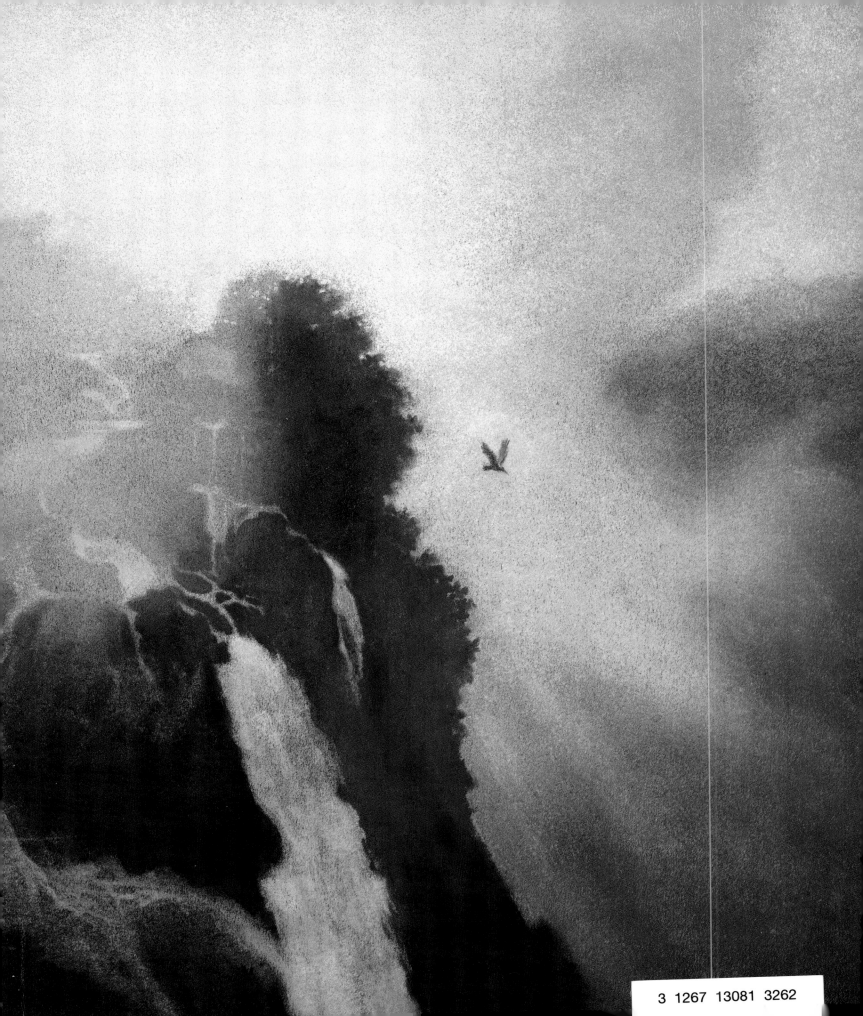

3 1267 13081 3262

TO MARGARET EMILY
——JH AND KB

FOR KAI
——FC

Oil wash on board was used for the full-color illustrations. The text type is 12-point Novarese Bold.

Text copyright © 1998 by James Haskins and Kathleen Benson
Illustrations copyright © 1998 by Floyd Cooper

All rights reserved. No part of this book may be reproduced or utilized in any form or by any means,
electronic or mechanical, including photocopying, recording, or by any information storage and retrieval system,
without permission in writing from the Publisher.

Published by Lothrop, Lee & Shepard Books
an imprint of Morrow Junior Books
a division of William Morrow and Company, Inc.
1350 Avenue of the Americas, New York, NY 10019
www.williammorrow.com

Printed in Singapore at Tien Wah Press.
Designed by Rachel Simon

1 2 3 4 5 6 7 8 9 10

Library of Congress Cataloging-in-Publication Data
Haskins, James.
African beginnings/by James Haskins and Kathleen Benson; illustrated by Floyd Cooper.
p. cm.
ISBN 0-688-10256-5 (trade)——ISBN 0-688-10257-3 (library)
1. Africa——History——Juvenile literature.  [1. Africa——History.]  1. Benson, Kathleen. II. Cooper, Floyd, ill. III. Title.
DT22.H323 1998   960-dc20   94-9848   CIP AC

With special thanks to Dr. John Henrik Clarke and Dr. Enid Schildkrout for their invaluable assistance.

# CONTENTS

# Ancient Africa

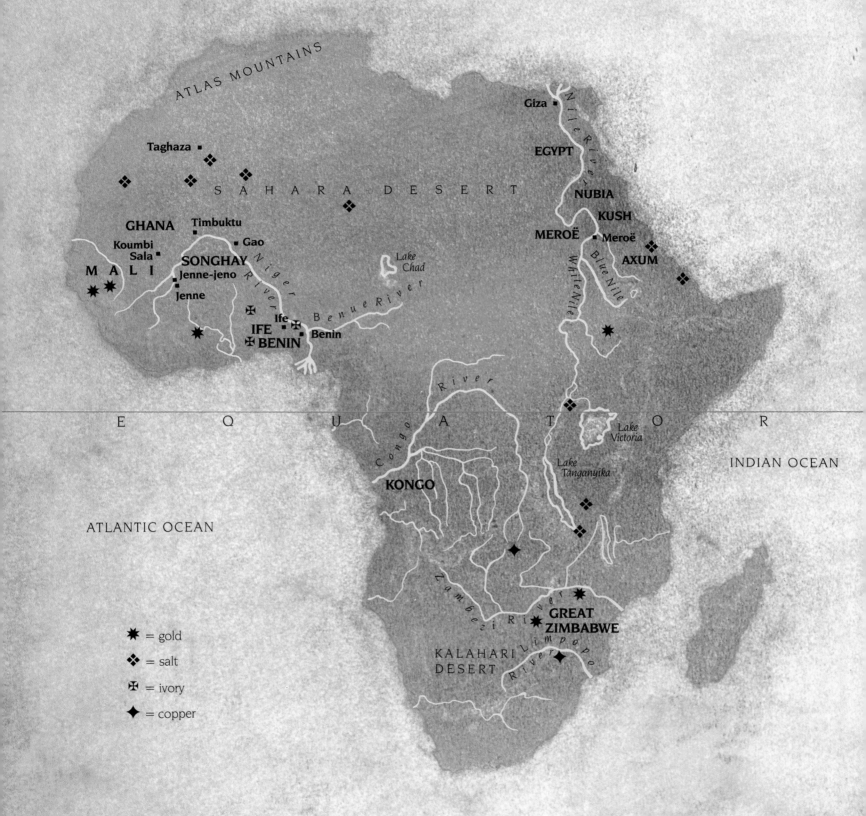

ATLAS MOUNTAINS

Giza ■

EGYPT

NUBIA

KUSH

MEROË ● Meroë ■

AXUM

SAHARA DESERT

Taghaza ■

GHANA

Timbuktu ■

Koumbi Sala ■

Gao ■

SONGHAY

MALI

Jenne-jeno ■

Jenne ■

Niger River

Benue River

Ife ■

IFE
BENIN

Benin ■

Lake Chad

Nile River

White Nile

Blue Nile

Congo River

E    Q    U    A    T    O    R

Lake Victoria

Lake Tanganyika

INDIAN OCEAN

KONGO

ATLANTIC OCEAN

Zambezi River

GREAT ZIMBABWE

KALAHARI DESERT

Limpopo River

✸ = gold

❖ = salt

✠ = ivory

◆ = copper

This map shows the general locations of the most important ancient African kingdoms and cities, which rose and fell in the period from 3800 B.C. to A.D. 1800. Territory and power ranged over time, with one empire often taking over another.

AFRICAN CIVILIZATION DATES BACK TO A TIME (BETWEEN TWELVE THOUSAND AND SEVEN thousand years ago) when the region called the Sahara—now a vast desert—was green and fertile. Shepherds and herdsmen of the Sahara and southern Africa developed advanced herding and agricultural methods that allowed them to live at more than a subsistence level. Some people became skilled in crafts, such as pottery. Others created rock art. Activities portrayed in rock art made some six thousand years ago—including fishing, hunting, and gathering—reflect the lives of the people in these communities. Tools of stone, bone, and wood also give insight into their lives. As the people prospered, they began to engage in trade with their neighbors, and some communities grew in size and power.

Many cultures thrived on this huge continent, from the ancient kingdoms of Egypt and Nubia to the great sub-Saharan (south of the Sahara) empires in what is now western Sudan to the forest kingdoms of central Africa. As the Sahara became dry, the northern and southern parts of the continent were divided by an arid region larger than the mainland of the United States. A community that lived by farming in the Nile River delta developed a way of life very different from that of a nomadic people who lived near the Sahara Desert or a society that mined gold, silver, or copper. But through trade and other forms of contact, these societies influenced one another. As with all civilizations, the development of African civilization did not proceed along a straight line, but in a much more complicated fashion, with various kingdoms growing out of one another, centers of invention existing in different places at the same time, and many more communities flourishing than can be reflected in this book.

Although writing existed in several of the ancient kingdoms, African history was generally based in spoken tradition. But art, architecture, and artifacts have provided us with some important clues about how people farmed and prepared food, worshiped, organized governments, developed natural resources, made scientific inquiries and calculations, and much more.

Much of Africa's past was ignored or misunderstood by the Europeans who arrived in the 1400s in search of trade routes to India. Their search led them to the treasures of Africa, and it was these treasures, not Africa's rich history, that occupied their minds. At first, these traders sought gold, ivory, and spices. Later, after European colonization in the New World of the Americas, European traders undertook a huge commerce in human lives. To exploit the riches of the New World, they purchased millions of Africans, forcing them to leave their families and homelands forever. The slaves who survived the brutal journey to the New World brought a legacy of African history and culture as rich and diverse as the continent itself.

Many clues to Africa's past are still waiting to be discovered, explored, and better understood. Although this book can show only a glimpse of Africa's fascinating history, it is a place to begin.

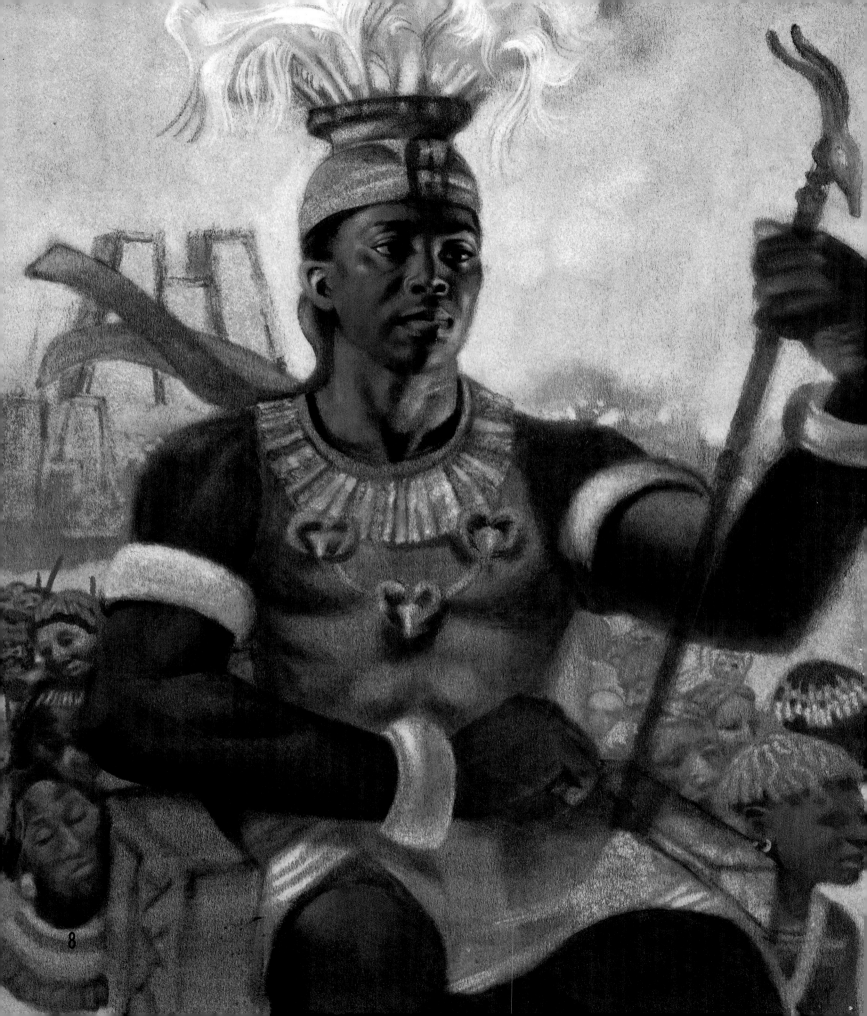

# NUBIA

ONE OF THE OLDEST AND WEALTHIEST OF ANCIENT AFRICAN CULTURES was Nubia, south of the Egyptian kingdom, in the area of present-day southern Egypt and northern Sudan. The Nubian culture, which began around 3800 B.C., had plentiful resources and used advanced farming methods. Nubia carried on a thriving business in gold (*nub* was the word for "gold" in Old Egyptian), ebony, cattle, ivory, ostrich plumes, and more. Egypt was Nubia's major trading partner, in both materials and ideas.

Many archaeologists argue that the idea of divine kingship (the belief that a ruler is a god in human form) originated in Nubia, even before it appeared in Egypt around 3100 B.C. The Nubians created elaborate tombs with many chambers for their kings. These great mounds of gravel were filled with whatever the dead might need in the afterlife—incense burners, mirrors, inscribed plaques, and magical figurines to serve them.

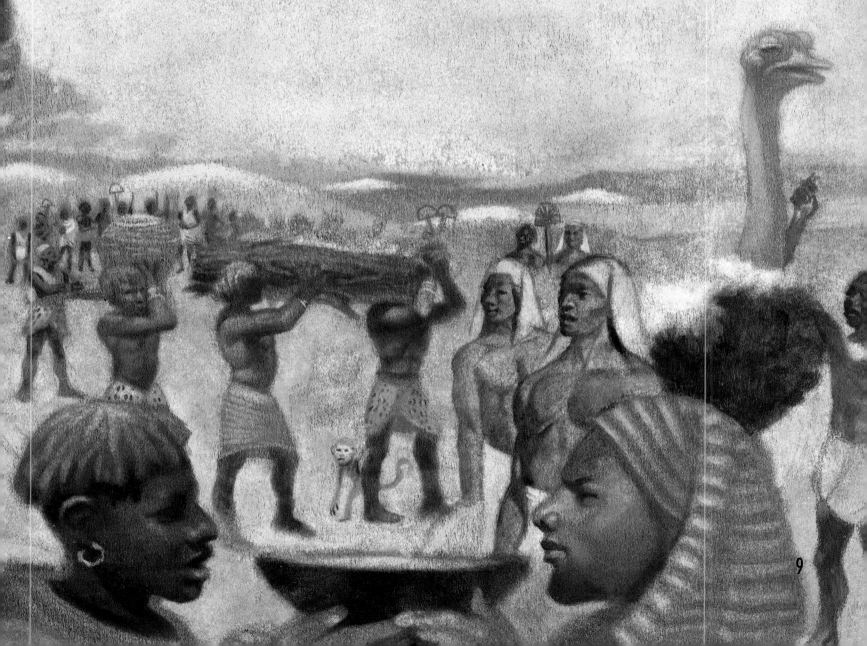

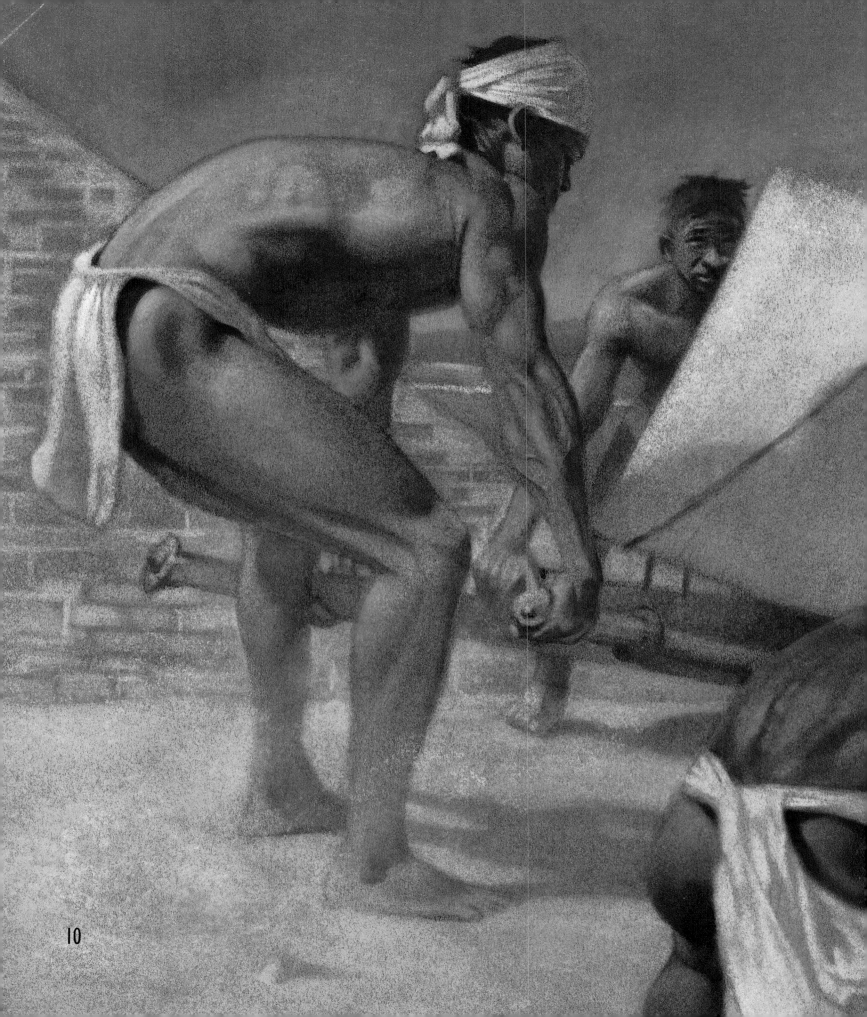

# EGYPT

MUCH MORE IS KNOWN ABOUT THE ANCIENT CULTURE OF EGYPT. THE FERTILE SOIL AROUND THE GREAT Nile River—the longest river in the world—was ideal for farming, and farming fostered the development of early civilization. By 3500 B.C., the Egyptians had formed states. Four hundred years later, Lower and Upper Egypt were unified, and a great civilization began. Around 3000 B.C., the Egyptians developed a system of writing (in symbols called hieroglyphs), enabling them to record their history and share their knowledge with one another.

Egypt is best known to us as the land of the pharaohs (divine kings) and of the huge pyramids that were built as their tombs. In about 2550 B.C., the pharaoh Khufu (Cheops) ordered the building of the Great Pyramid at Giza, one of the largest structures ever built. The set of solid limestone blocks covers thirteen acres, and the base is a square, seven hundred fifty-six feet on each side. It may have taken ten years to build the access roads for the pyramid's construction and the underground burial chambers below the base, then another twenty years to build the pyramid itself.

Stones for the body of the pyramid were quarried at Jebel Mokattam, which is in present-day Cairo. The facing stones were brought from the southeast, near present-day Aswân. The massive stones were dragged to the Nile and carried by barges to Giza; then, with levers and ramps, they were transported uphill to the pyramid site. Thousands of laborers worked on the construction every day.

The Egyptians constructed about seventy pyramids over fifteen hundred years. The Great Pyramid was the tallest ever built. Such enormous projects required extensive engineering, construction, mathematical, and administrative skills.

Even tombs as large as the pyramids, however, could not prevent the decay of the bodies buried within them. So Egyptian scientists put their minds to discovering a method of preservation. Between 2500 and 2000 B.C., they invented the mummification process: a way of preserving dead bodies by treating them with special chemicals and wrapping them in layers of cloth.

11

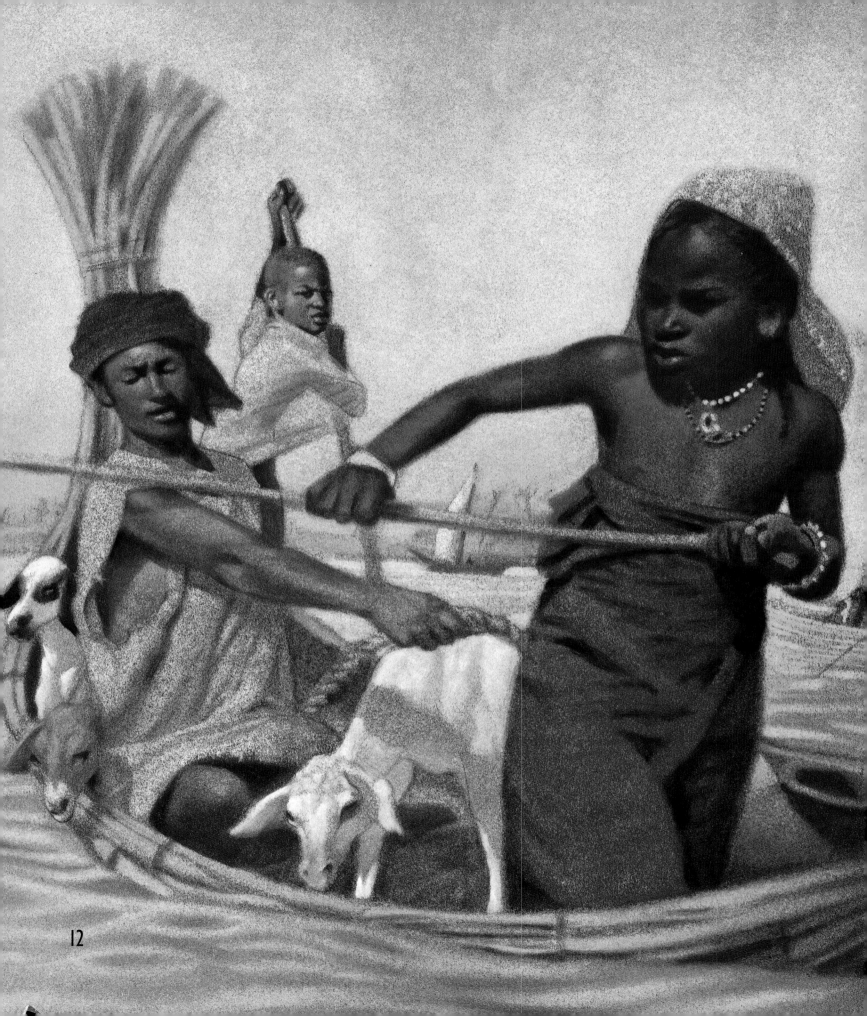

Egyptians sailed the Nile River on trading expeditions. Carrying incense, ebony, grain, and ivory, they traveled south to exchange their goods for gold and slaves. In this way, they traded with the Nubians, as well as with the people of the kingdom of Kush, south of Nubia. The Egyptians later brought the Nubians and the Kushites under their control, but eventually they were taken over themselves for a century by the Kushites.

The mighty Nile was not only a remarkable trade route and a spur to civilization, it was also the source of Egypt's agricultural strength. Its annual flooding was critically important for farming. In order to calculate when to expect the floods, Egyptians studied the sun, moon, and stars, and in the process developed the world's first known twelve-month calendar of three hundred sixty-five days.

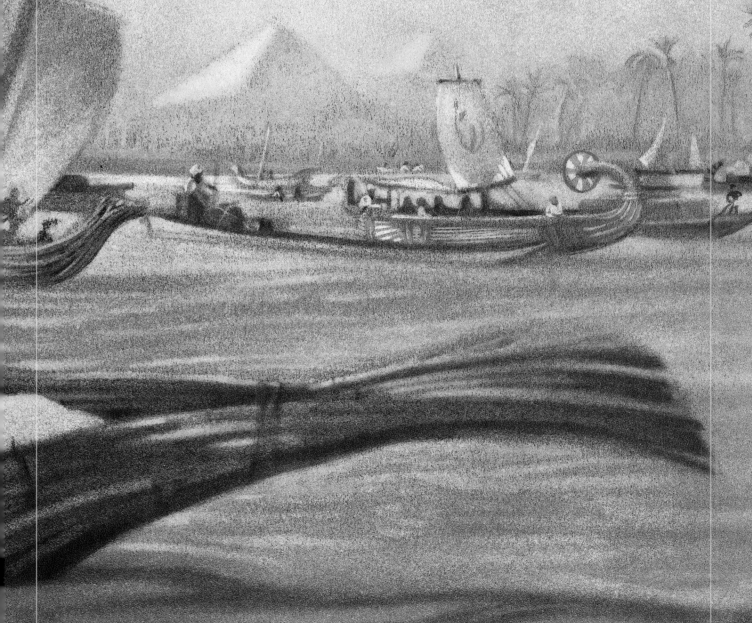

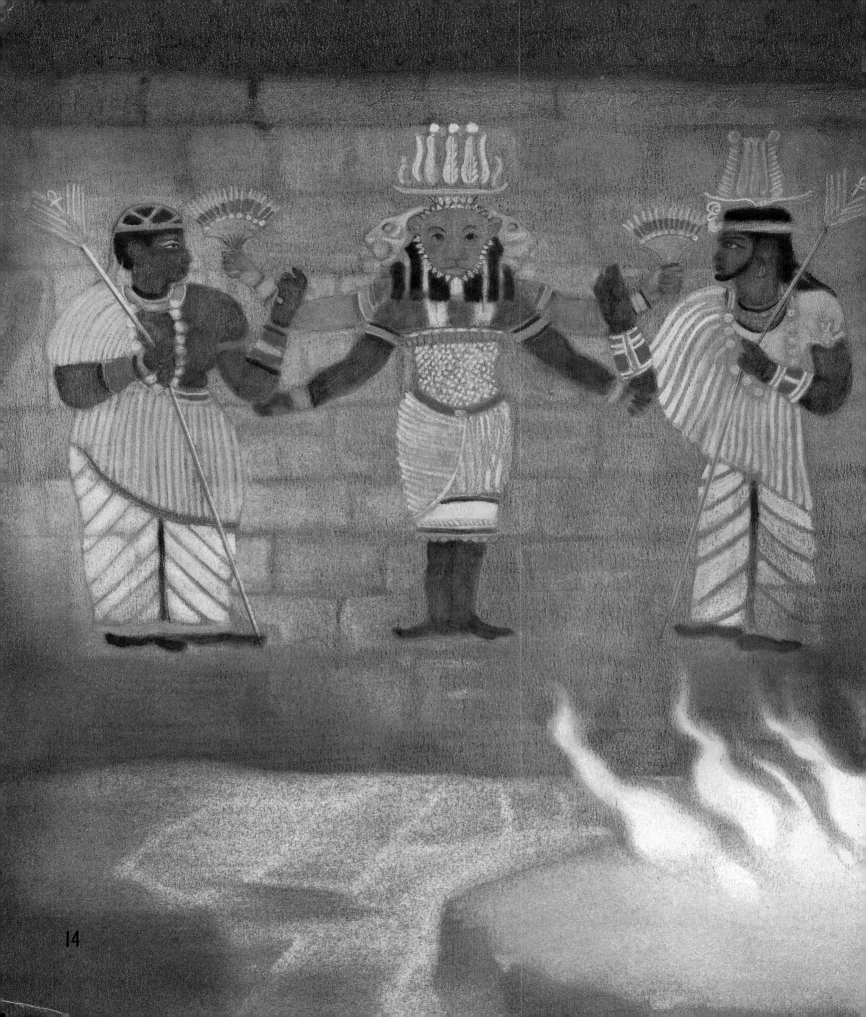

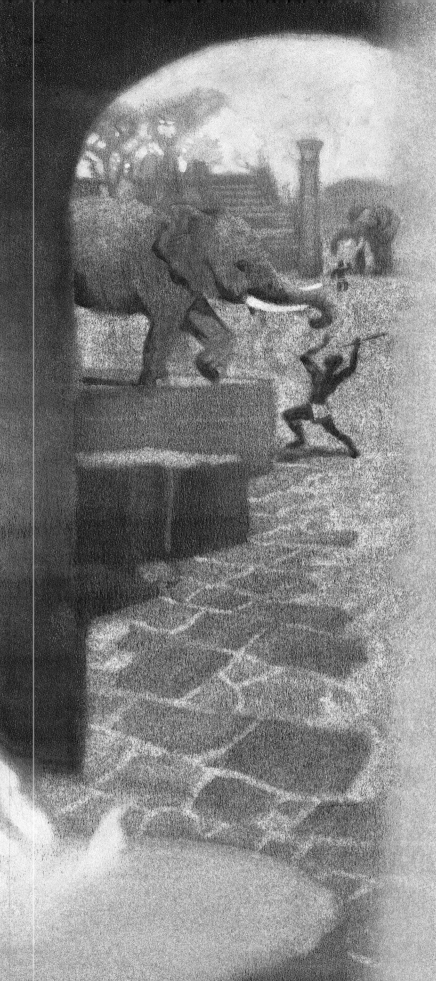

# KUSH AND MEROË

SOUTH OF NUBIA AND EGYPT WAS THE KINGDOM of Kush, a very old civilization that enjoyed a resurgence beginning around 900 B.C. For nearly a century, from about 750 B.C., the Kushite kings ruled Egypt. These kings are shown in Egyptian temple and tomb depictions as black pharaohs. The Kushite reign ended when Assyrian armies conquered Egypt. From the sixth century B.C. onward, the Kushite kings ruled their territory from the population center of Meroë, farther down the Nile.

Ruled by goddess-queens and god-kings, Meroë became a powerful empire by 100 B.C. It was renowned as an industrial center where local ore was mined, smelted, and forged into iron. The Meroitic culture may have helped to spread iron technology to other parts of Africa. The Kushites in Meroë developed their own system of writing, which has yet to be deciphered by modern scholars.

The Kushites traveled widely, and their civilization at Meroë was known for its distinctive art, architecture, and sense of enterprise. Even their use of animals was unusual: They domesticated elephants for military use and for impressive display.

Meroë eventually was overshadowed by Axum, its nearest neighbor. By A.D. 350, Meroë was part of the Axumite Empire, which covered what is now northern Ethiopia.

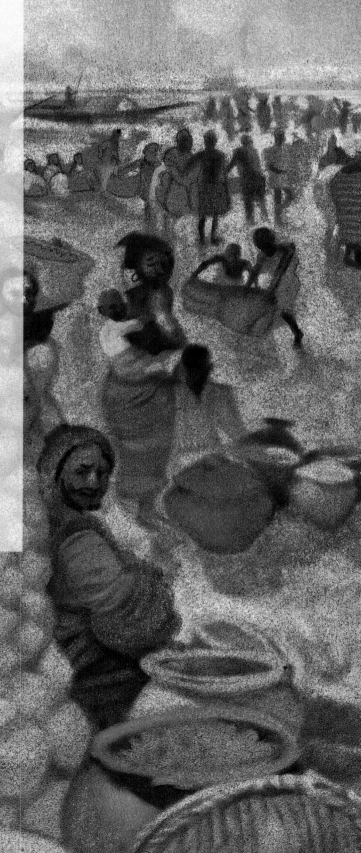

# JENNE-JENO

IN THE INLAND DELTA REGION of the present-day Republic of Mali in West Africa, the first known city south of the Sahara arose in a fertile land where the Bani and Niger Rivers flow. Jenne-jeno was an urban center whose advanced culture was marked by productive agriculture, elegant craftsmanship, and far-reaching trade. Established—probably by herders and fishermen—as a small group of round mud huts around 250 B.C., by A.D. 800 Jenne-jeno was a cosmopolitan center of some ten thousand people, surrounded by a massive mud-brick wall some ten feet wide and thirteen or more feet in height.

The people of Jenne-jeno traded first with the Timbuktu region downriver and later, by caravan, with North Africa. In exchange for Saharan salt and copper and Mediterranean glass beads, the merchants of Jenne-jeno offered an abundance of crafts, including gold and copper jewelry, as well as such agricultural produce as red rice, onions, and chili peppers. The oldest gold earring yet found in West Africa was found in excavations at Jenne-jeno, along with pottery burial urns and toys in the shape of animals.

Around A.D. 1400, Jenne-jeno was abandoned, and in the centuries since, oral histories relating to it disappeared, leaving the reason for its abandonment a mystery. A new city named Jenne arose about two miles away. It grew and prospered as a rich center for agricultural exports, and continues as such today.

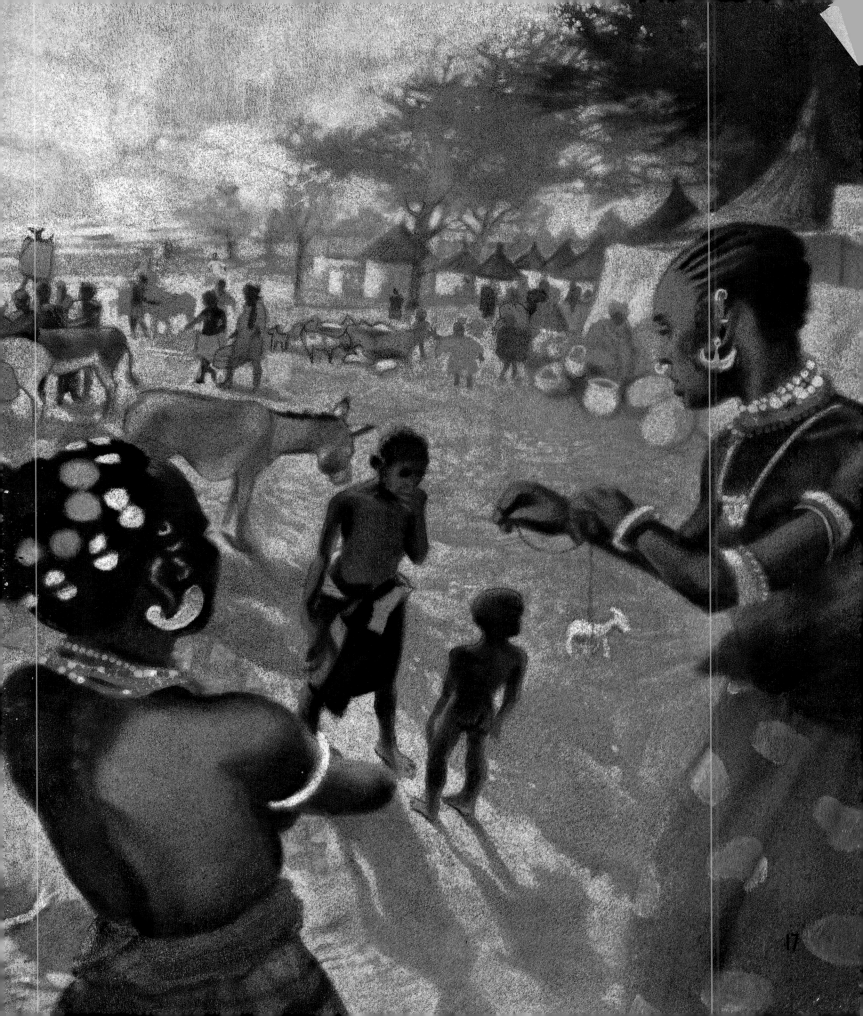

17

# THE SPREAD OF ISLAM

NORTH AFRICAN ARABS traveled south to trade. They first sailed down the eastern coast of the continent, and by the seventh century they had begun crossing the vast Sahara Desert with caravans of camels to trade for African gold, silver, copper, ivory, pepper, kola nuts, salt, and slaves. In exchange, they brought spearheads and axes, glass, wine, and wheat. They also brought their religion, Islam.

Founded by Muhammad (who lived from about A.D. 570 to 632), the religion of Islam is based on the belief in one God, Allah, and on a life of devotion to Allah by the faithful. One of the most important duties of a Muslim, a believer in Islam, is to spread the faith, and Arabs went southward in ever-increasing numbers to settle in the African population centers and bring Islam to the people there. The religion of Islam allows for great diversity, so it was possible for Africans to adopt Islam and still keep many of their traditional ways.

The Arabs introduced not only their religion but also their systems of currency and credit, their administrative structure, their political ideas, and their language and writing. Many accounts of African history were written in Arabic script.

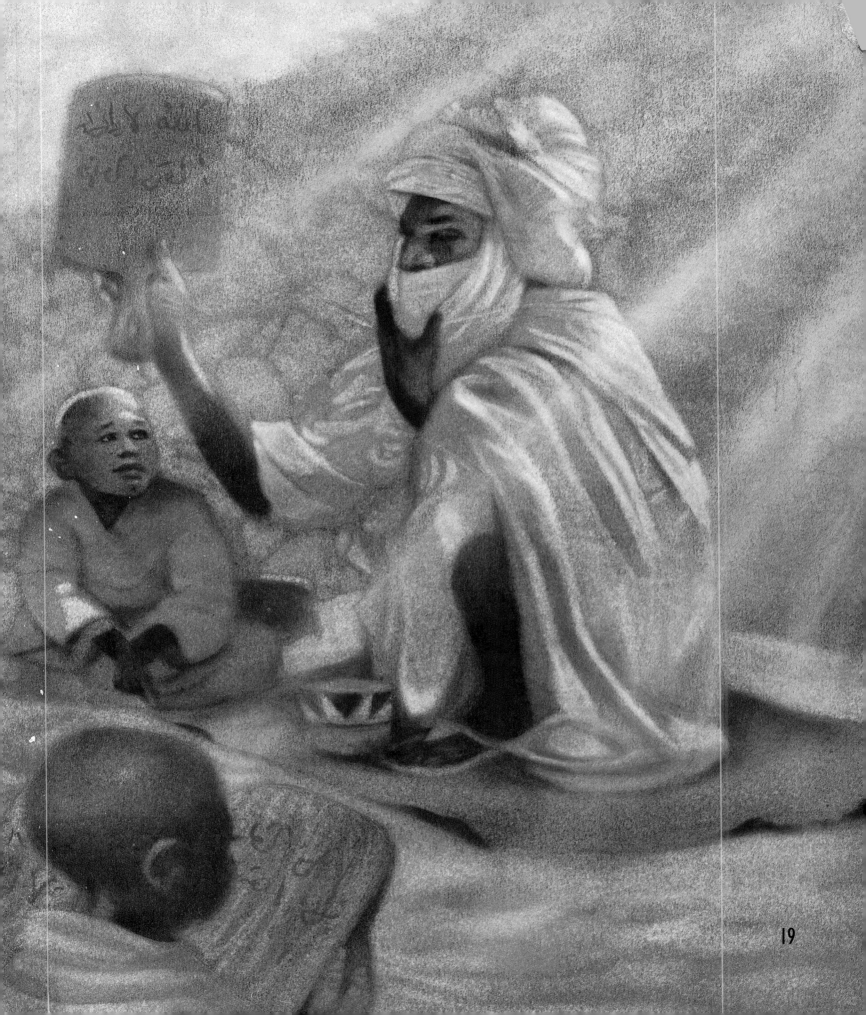

# GHANA

WHEN GREAT NUMBERS OF ARAB CAMEL CARAVANS STARTED TO CROSS THE SAHARA to trade, the West African kingdom of Ghana began to strengthen its power. Founded in the fifth century A.D., Ghana soon established itself as a center of the iron industry. When the trans-Saharan trade began to flourish, so too did Ghana, by taxing and monitoring the trade. Gold arrived from secret locations in the south, and between about A.D. 450 and 1230, more gold was traded in Ghana than anywhere else in the world. Salt—a vital commodity as a food preservative—came from the north, chiefly from the mines at Taghaza, in the Sahara.

The people of the original kingdom, the Soninkes, spoke the Mande language. In Mande, *ghana* means "warrior king," and the Soninkes were true to the name. They took over other kingdoms, and Ghana became an empire that covered most of the territory between the Niger River and the Atlantic Ocean.

At its height, in A.D. 1060, the empire influenced the territory of present-day Senegal, Mauritania, and Mali. Arab travelers described an imperial army of two hundred thousand soldiers, including forty thousand archers. Since many diverse cultures were incorporated into Ghana, the chief ruler had to have a strong system of justice and administration to keep peace in the empire.

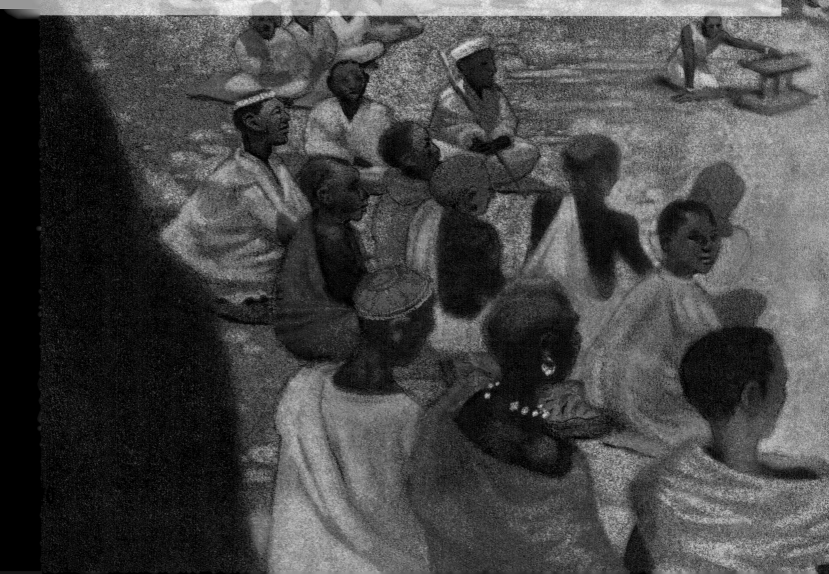

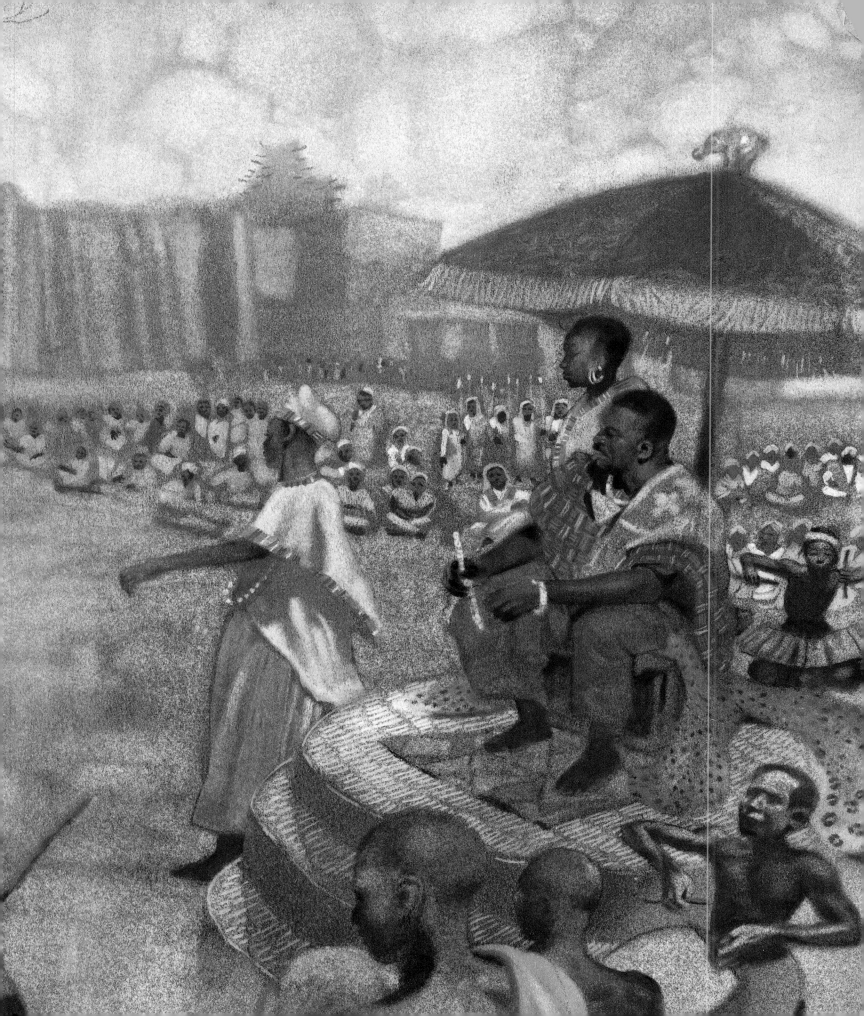

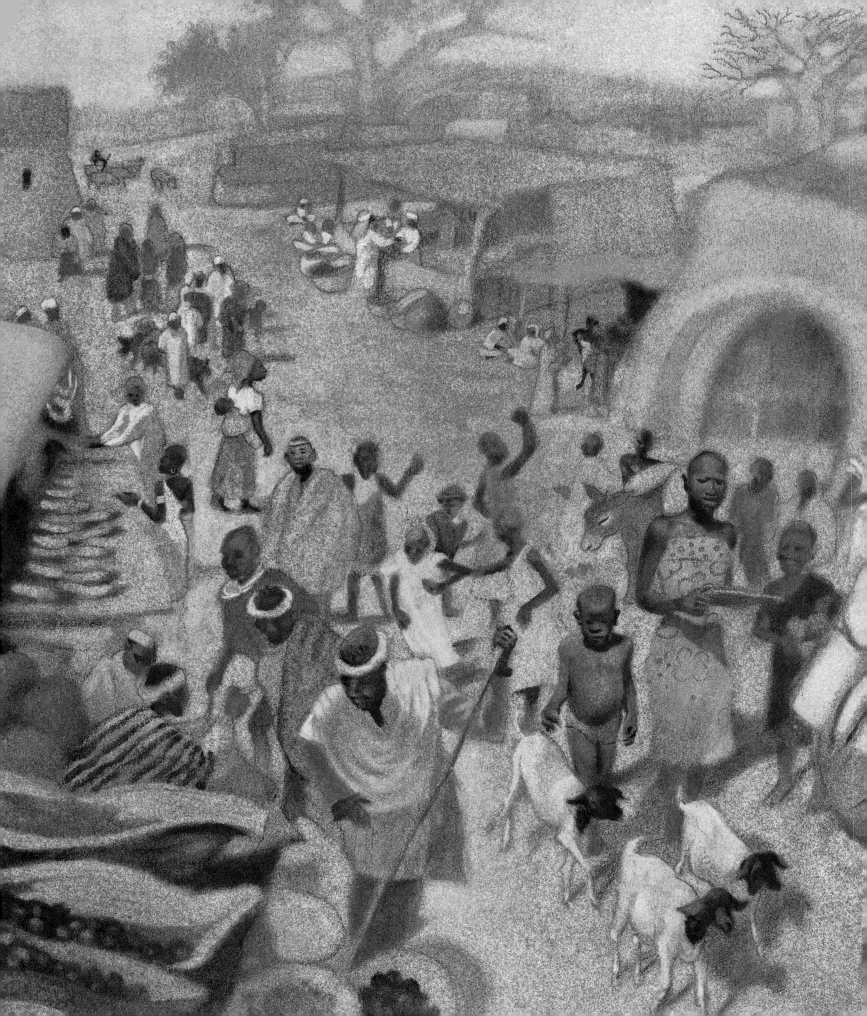

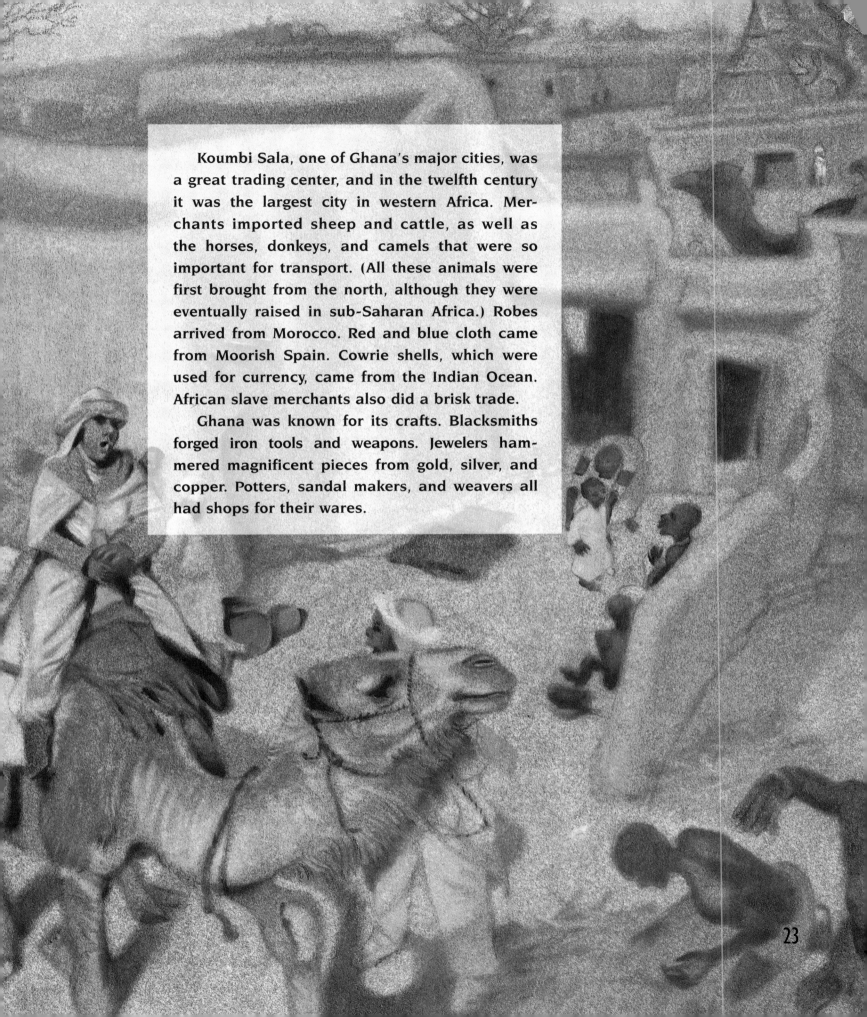

Koumbi Sala, one of Ghana's major cities, was a great trading center, and in the twelfth century it was the largest city in western Africa. Merchants imported sheep and cattle, as well as the horses, donkeys, and camels that were so important for transport. (All these animals were first brought from the north, although they were eventually raised in sub-Saharan Africa.) Robes arrived from Morocco. Red and blue cloth came from Moorish Spain. Cowrie shells, which were used for currency, came from the Indian Ocean. African slave merchants also did a brisk trade.

Ghana was known for its crafts. Blacksmiths forged iron tools and weapons. Jewelers hammered magnificent pieces from gold, silver, and copper. Potters, sandal makers, and weavers all had shops for their wares.

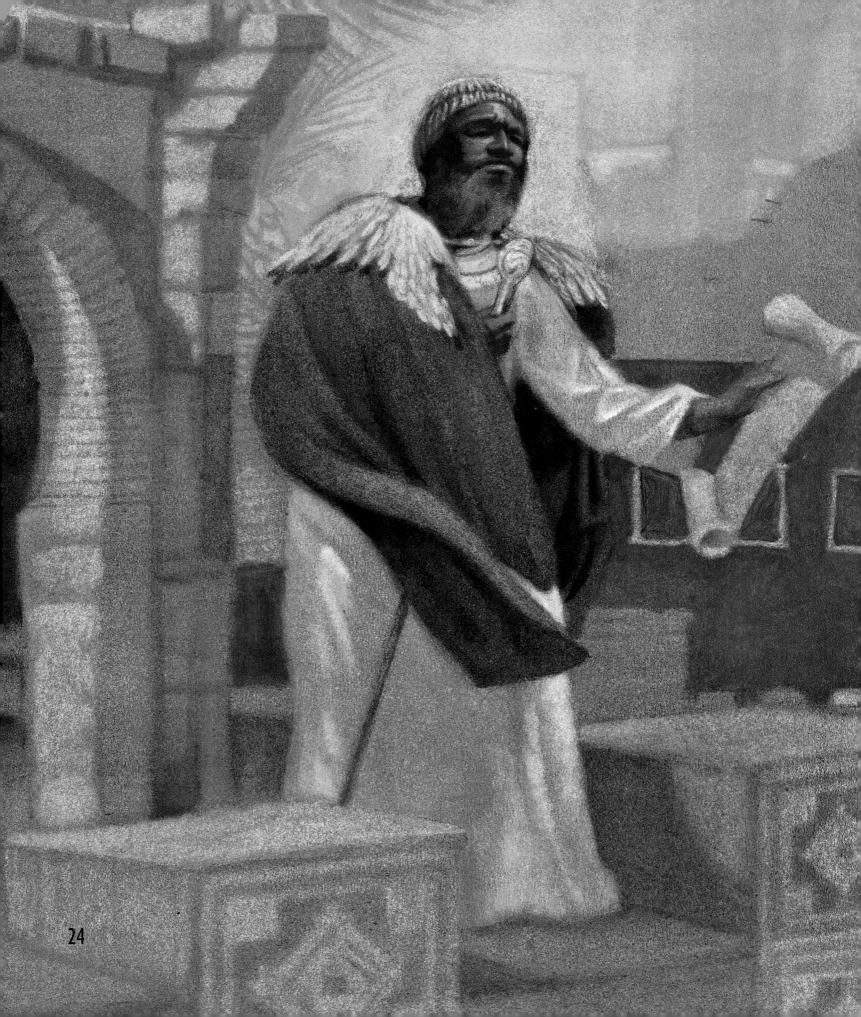

# MALI

IN THE THIRTEENTH CENTURY A.D., THE MANDINKA PEOPLE OF THE STATE of Kangaba emerged as successors to the Ghanaian rulers. Their Islamic emperor, Mansa Musa, came to the throne in 1312 and died in 1337. During his reign, the Mandinka began to gain control over Ghana's gold trade, and the empire of Mali overtook that of Ghana.

Mansa Musa oversaw more than conquests and trade. He also had a great influence on architecture in his empire. While on a pilgrimage to Mecca (in present-day Saudi Arabia), he was impressed by the architectural styles he saw, and he brought back an architect to design new Muslim mosques. Although sun-dried mud bricks had long been used for building, Mansa Musa introduced a new building style that combined the mud bricks with timber beams. This style of building made possible the construction of multistory houses.

The Mali Empire was so significant that nations as far off as southern Europe recognized its power. A map of Africa prepared in 1375 by cartographer Abraham Cresques on Majorca (an island off the coast of Spain) depicted the emperor of Mali seated majestically upon a throne while traders from North Africa approached his markets.

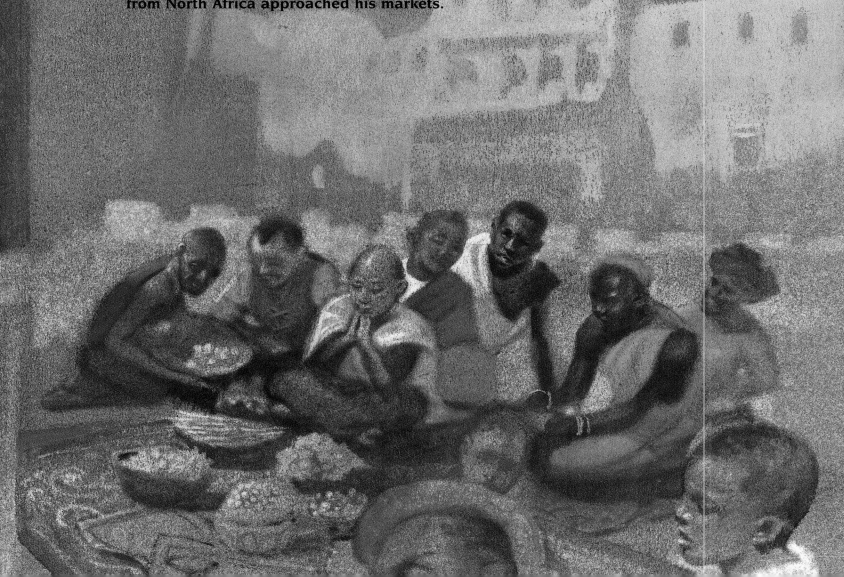

# SONGHAY

AROUND THE EIGHTH OR NINTH CENTURY A.D., the Songhay people occupied Gao, the most important city on the Middle Niger River south of Timbuktu, and began to build an empire of their own. In 1464, under the Muslim ruler Sonni Ali, the Songhay began the systematic conquest of their neighbors. They gained possession of Timbuktu and eventually controlled an area from the modern-day nation of Mali to what is now Nigeria. Their holdings included the third major city along the Niger, Jenne, which under the kingdom of Songhay continued to be one of the most important cities in Africa, with a noted university and medical school.

The Songhay civilization was highly organized. Everyone in the kingdom, including slaves, had obligations. Although slavery has never existed without some cruelty, African slaves were often treated as junior members of the community. In 1493, the new emperor, Askia Muhammad, inherited from his predecessor slaves whose obligations were to provide certain goods and services. Blacksmiths had to provide spears, fishermen had to deliver fish or canoes, cattle breeders had to bring in cattle, and others had to perform household services.

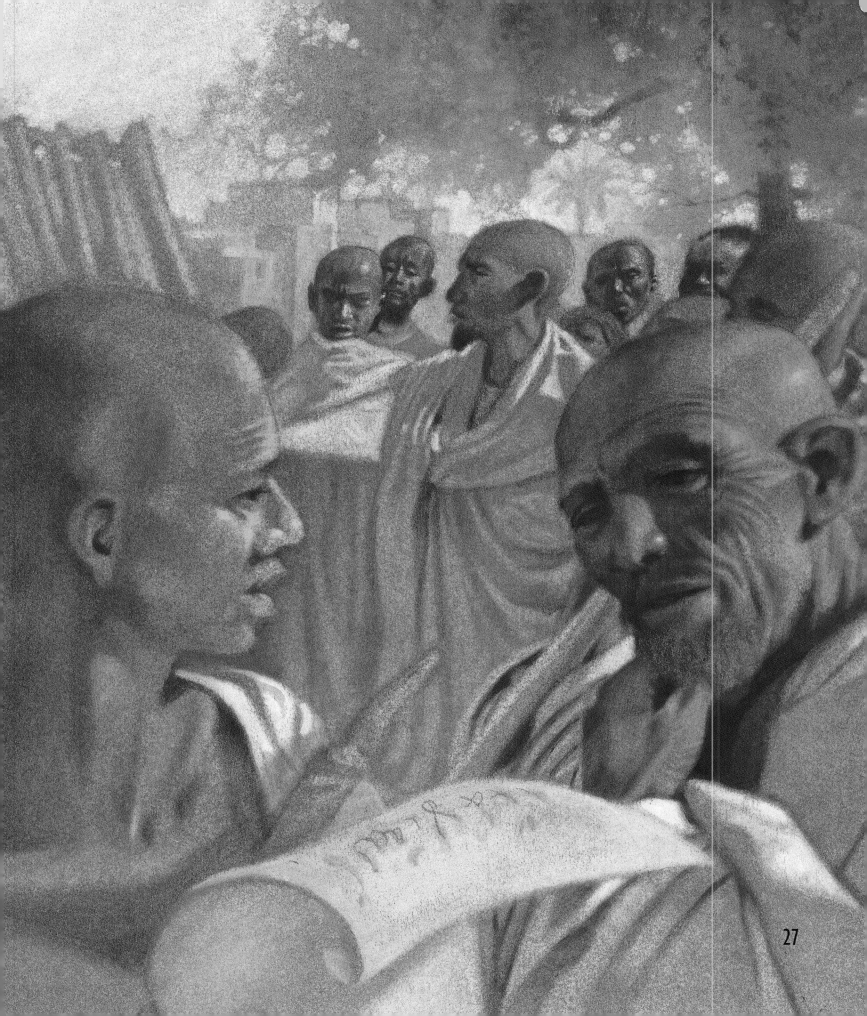

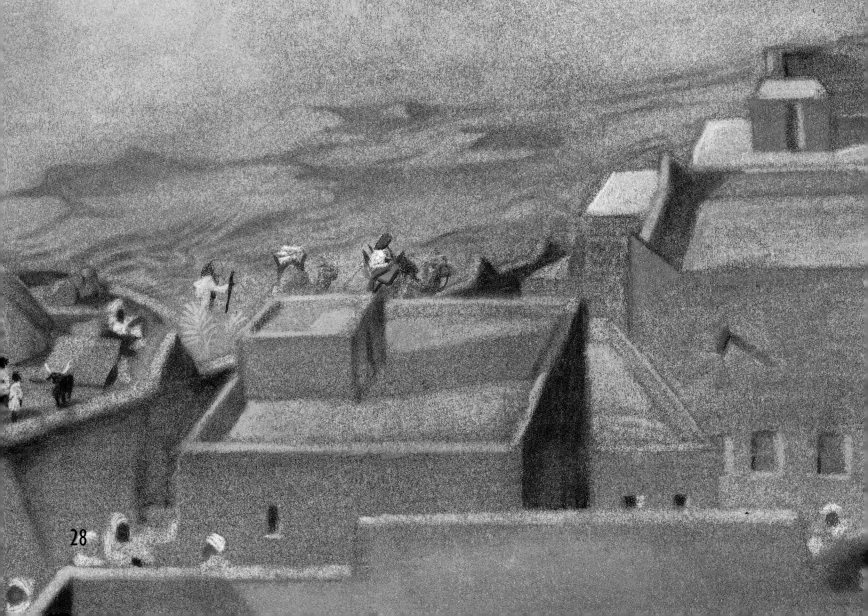

# TIMBUKTU

ASKIA MUHAMMAD UPHELD THE TRADITION OF ISLAMIC learning, and during his reign the university of Sankor thrived. Scholars from near and far were allowed to study, teach, and learn in Timbuktu, Gao, and Jenne.

By the late 1400s, the city of Timbuktu reflected the power of the Songhay. Arab travelers of the time described the crowded metropolis, with its markets, mosques, and impressive stone palace, as a resplendent capital of affluence and education.

In 1529, Askia Muhammad, more than eighty years old, was deposed by his son. In 1591, Morocco invaded and conquered the kingdom, effectively ending its influence.

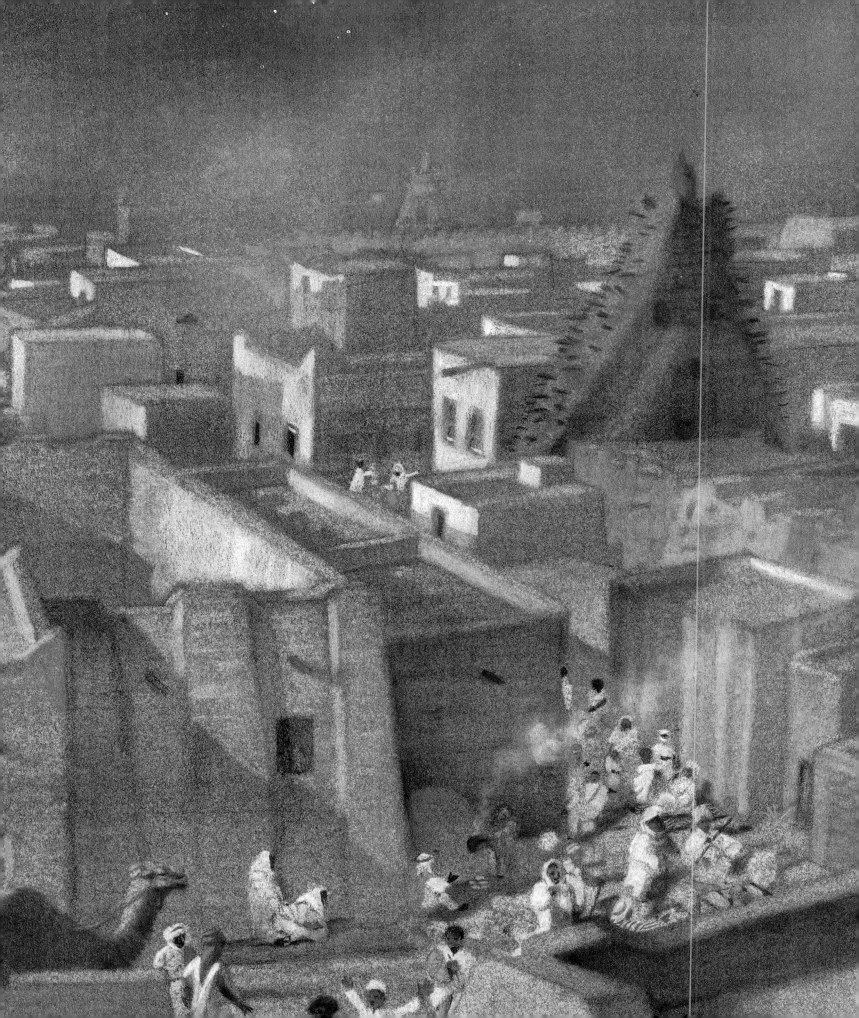

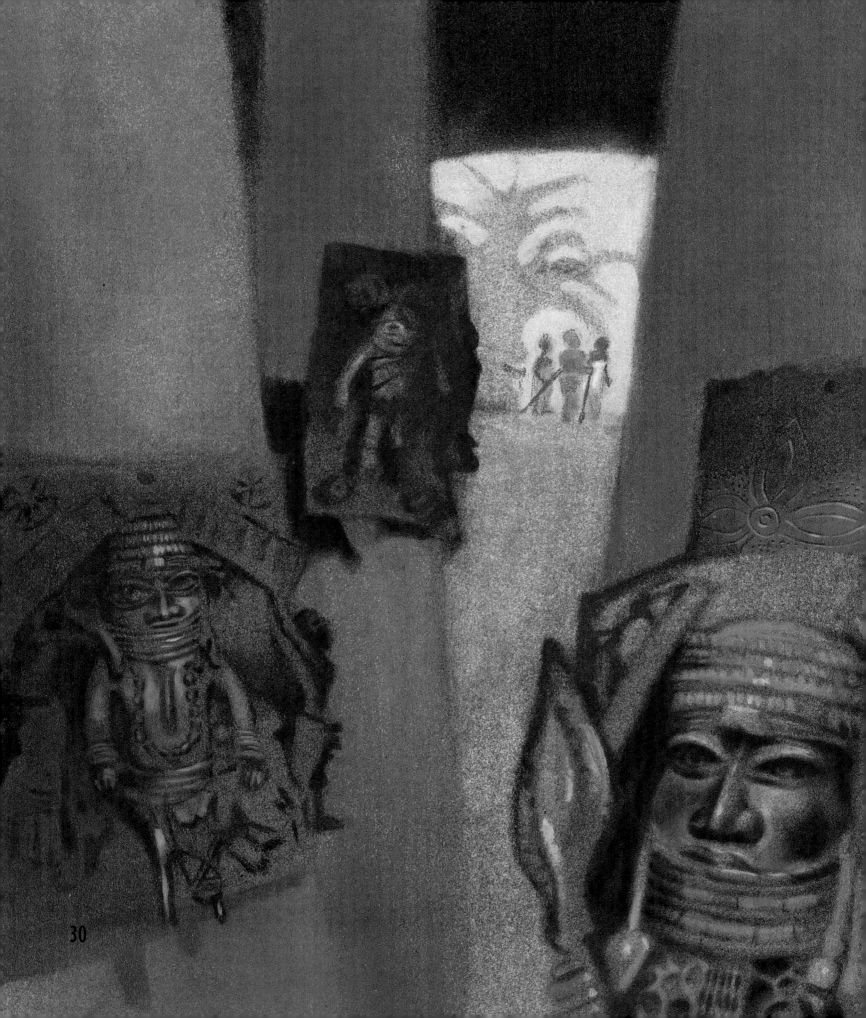

# BENIN

THE KINGDOM OF BENIN WAS located south of Songhay, in the forested delta area of the Niger and Benue Rivers in what is now southern Nigeria. It was established by the Yoruba people. Earlier, those same people had founded Ife, which in Yoruba lore was considered the place of creation, since it was there that Oduduwa, the mythical founder of the Yoruba people, established his throne.

The craftsmen of the ancient city-state of Ife created fine terra-cotta sculptures between the eleventh and fourteenth centuries A.D. Bronze castings of the heads of kings unearthed at the site of Ife in modern times reveal a technology more advanced than that in use in Europe during the same period.

Benin, both the kingdom and the capital city of the same name, emerged in the thirteenth century and peaked in the fifteenth. Like Ife, one of Benin's most important crafts was bronze casting, and some beautiful examples dating to the fifteenth and sixteenth centuries have been found. Benin bronzes could be distributed only by the *oba*, the divine king. Benin was famous as well for its jewelry makers, who worked in gold and ivory.

European traders arrived in Benin in the fifteenth century. Often motivated by the need for spices that would preserve food and enhance its flavor, they soon became more interested in ivory and slaves.

Portuguese traders described the metropolis of Benin as the grandest city in all of western Africa. Its houses were made of red clay polished to such a high luster that it looked like marble. Bronze plaques with scenes commemorating heroic deeds and events in the history of the people of Benin adorned pillars in the square galleries of the palaces.

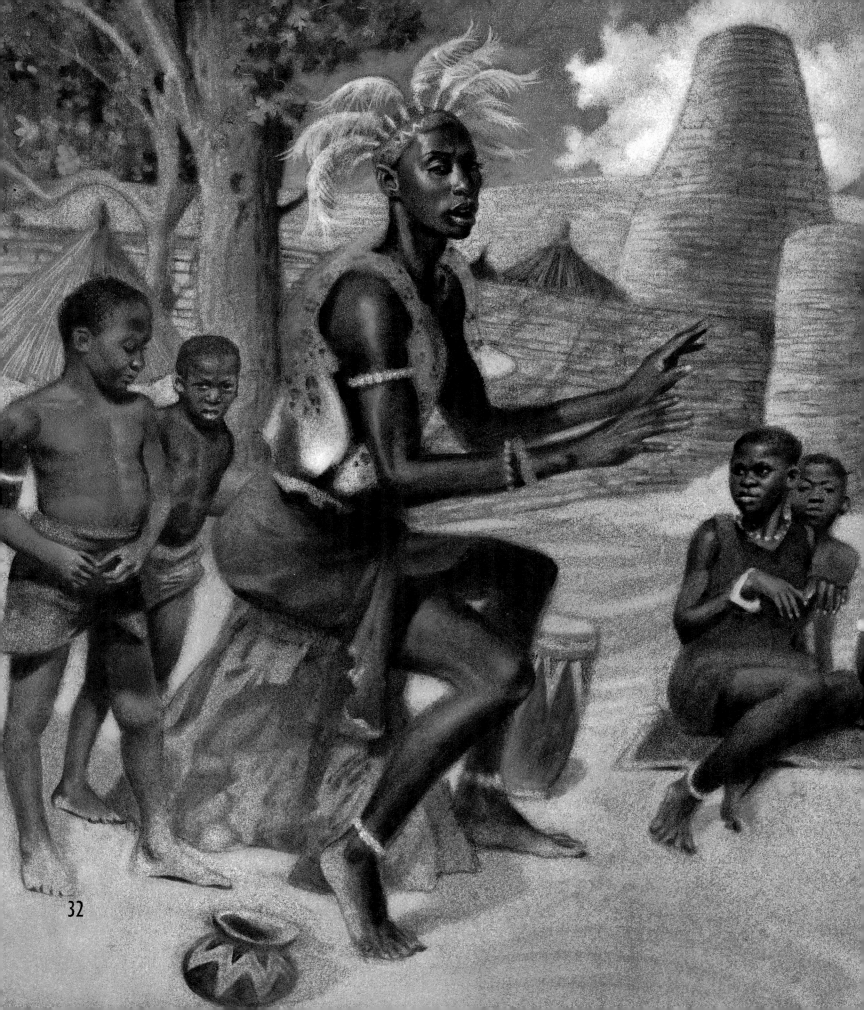

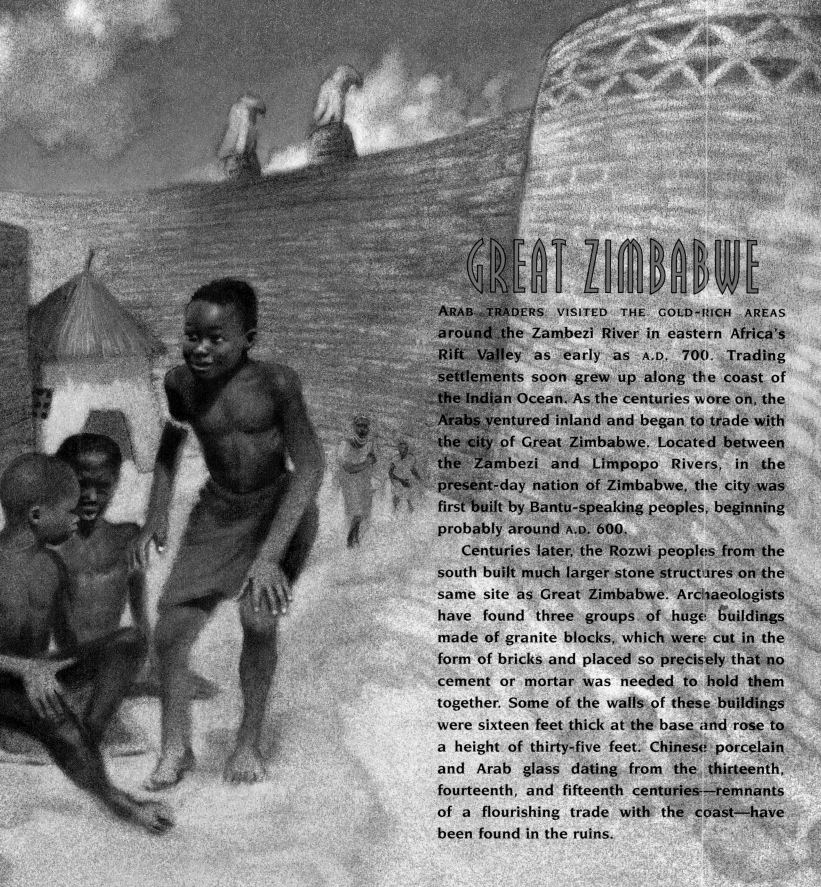

# GREAT ZIMBABWE

ARAB TRADERS VISITED THE GOLD-RICH AREAS around the Zambezi River in eastern Africa's Rift Valley as early as A.D. 700. Trading settlements soon grew up along the coast of the Indian Ocean. As the centuries wore on, the Arabs ventured inland and began to trade with the city of Great Zimbabwe. Located between the Zambezi and Limpopo Rivers, in the present-day nation of Zimbabwe, the city was first built by Bantu-speaking peoples, beginning probably around A.D. 600.

Centuries later, the Rozwi peoples from the south built much larger stone structures on the same site as Great Zimbabwe. Archaeologists have found three groups of huge buildings made of granite blocks, which were cut in the form of bricks and placed so precisely that no cement or mortar was needed to hold them together. Some of the walls of these buildings were sixteen feet thick at the base and rose to a height of thirty-five feet. Chinese porcelain and Arab glass dating from the thirteenth, fourteenth, and fifteenth centuries—remnants of a flourishing trade with the coast—have been found in the ruins.

33

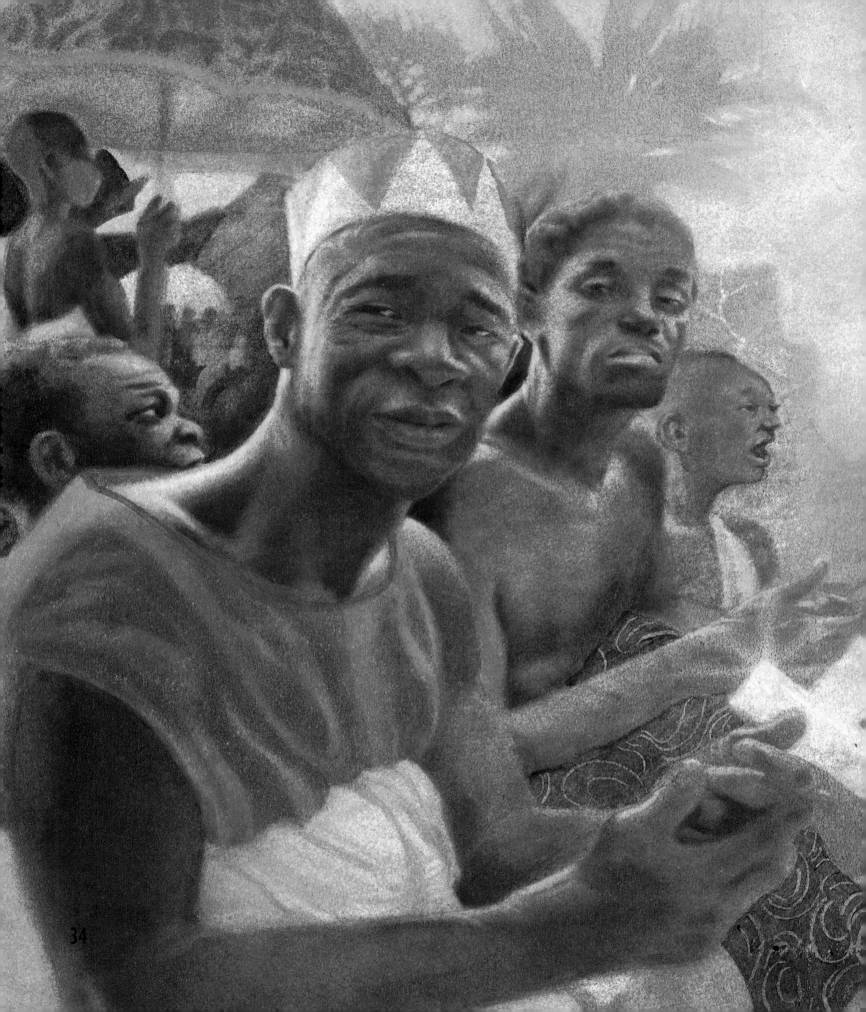

# KONGO

THE EMPIRE OF THE KONGO IN CENTRAL AFRICA, DATING TO THE fourteenth century, was known for a strong government and excellent craftsmanship. The empire was ruled by the *manikongo*, or king, and was divided into six provinces, each under a governor appointed by the king. Like most other powerful states, Kongo was a trading center. In the 1600s, the enormous amounts of cloth sold through the Kongo—over one hundred thousand yards to Africa alone—were comparable to the amounts sold by major textile-producing cities in Europe.

Kongo began a period of thriving commerce with Europe after Portuguese traders arrived in the 1480s. By 1491, Portuguese craftsmen, missionaries, and soldiers had settled in Mbanza, the capital. Afonso I, who became *manikongo* in 1505, was converted to Christianity by the Portuguese.

Afonso I had wide-reaching power. In 1525, for example, he ordered the seizure of a French ship and crew, declaring that they were sailing along the Kongo coast illegally. Both Afonso and his successor decided to call a temporary halt to the trade in slaves to other parts of Africa and overseas.

In 1641, *manikongo* Garcia II joined forces with the Dutch to control Portuguese slave traders, but the strong empire was ending. Twenty-four years later, Portuguese armies defeated the Kongo rulers and took control of the economy, which then became steadily weaker.

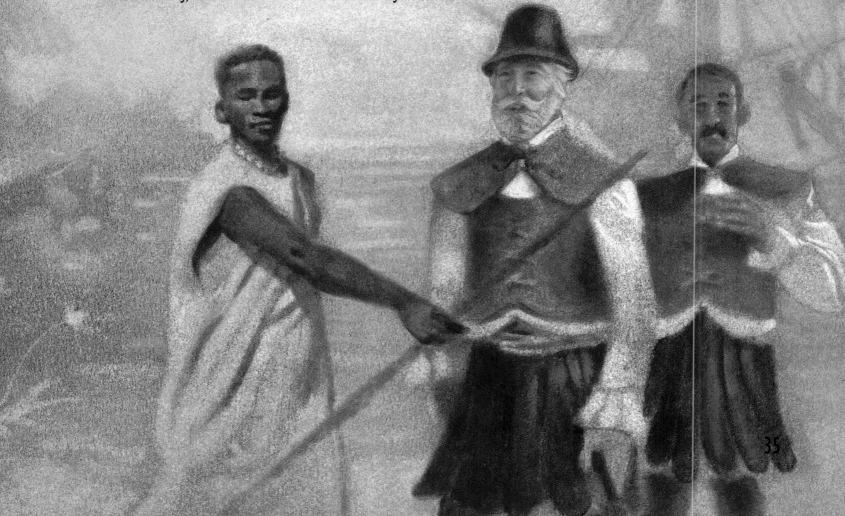

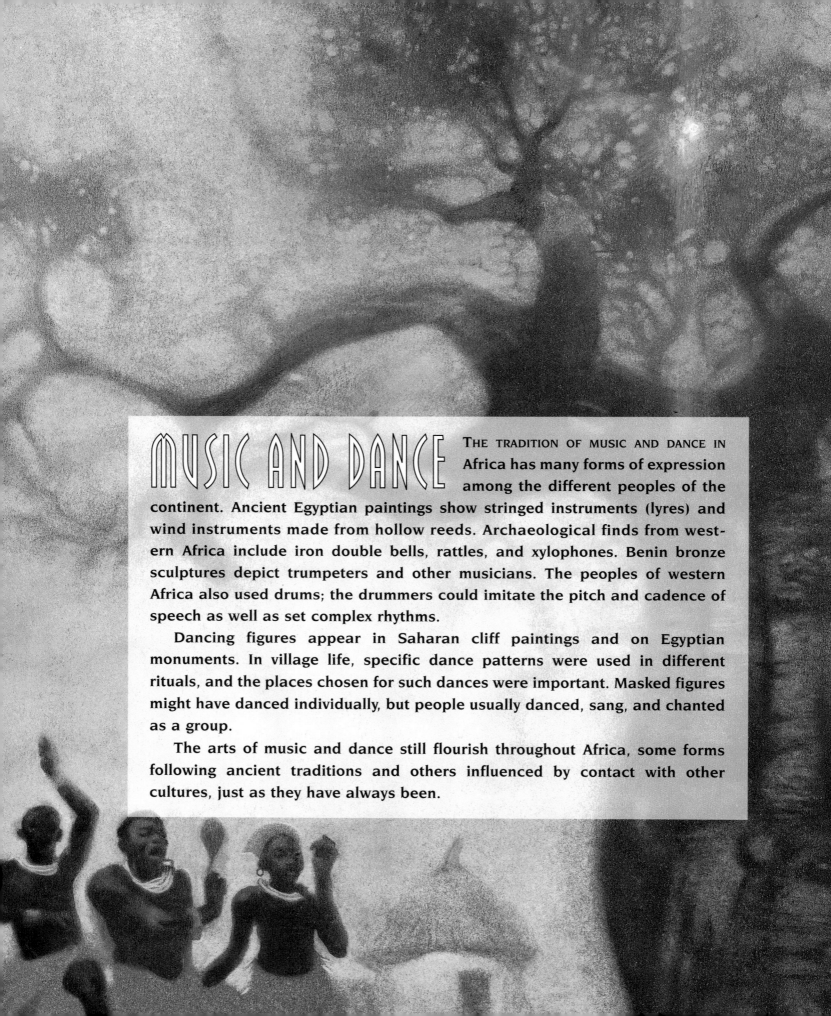

# MUSIC AND DANCE

THE TRADITION OF MUSIC AND DANCE IN Africa has many forms of expression among the different peoples of the continent. Ancient Egyptian paintings show stringed instruments (lyres) and wind instruments made from hollow reeds. Archaeological finds from western Africa include iron double bells, rattles, and xylophones. Benin bronze sculptures depict trumpeters and other musicians. The peoples of western Africa also used drums; the drummers could imitate the pitch and cadence of speech as well as set complex rhythms.

Dancing figures appear in Saharan cliff paintings and on Egyptian monuments. In village life, specific dance patterns were used in different rituals, and the places chosen for such dances were important. Masked figures might have danced individually, but people usually danced, sang, and chanted as a group.

The arts of music and dance still flourish throughout Africa, some forms following ancient traditions and others influenced by contact with other cultures, just as they have always been.

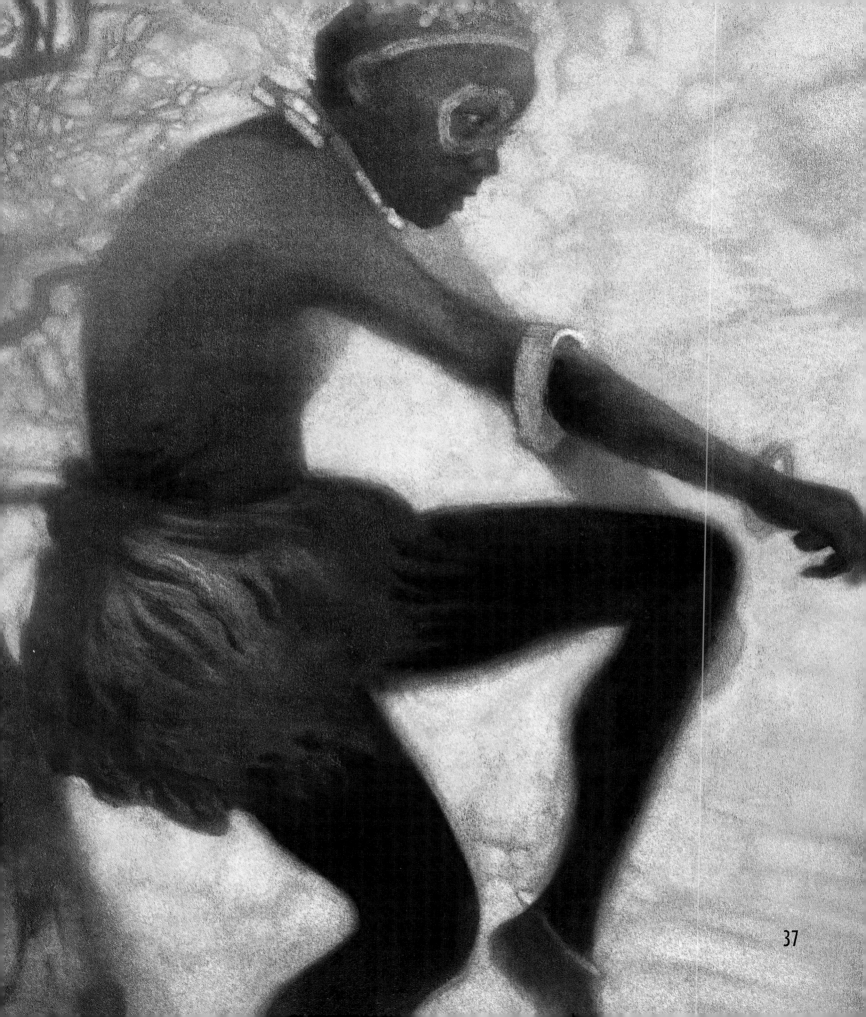

37

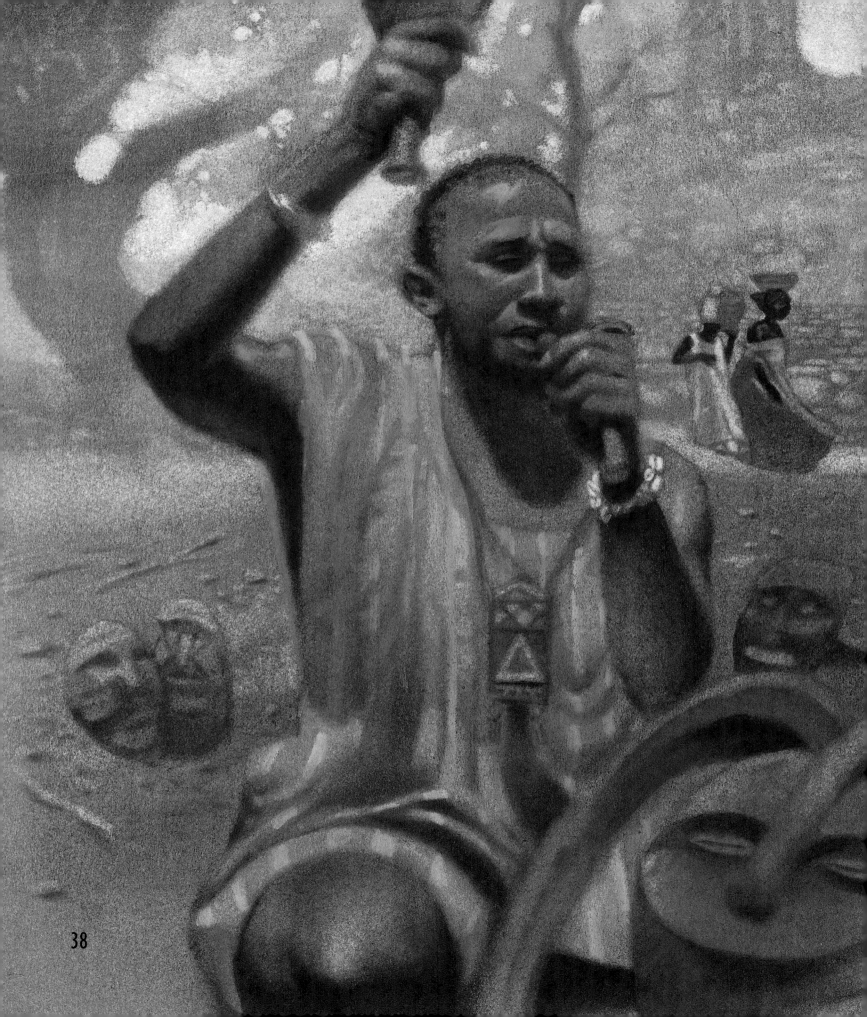

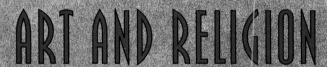

# ART AND RELIGION

LONG BEFORE THE SPREAD OF ISLAM AND Christianity, each of the many different African societies had its own religious system, based on the group's view of the place of humans in nature. Hunting peoples focused on the power of the forest and on spirits of animals; farming peoples on the importance of fertile land and the cycles of the seasons; and herding peoples on strong beliefs in sky-gods. All recognized the power of ancestors and their ties to others in the society. Some societies were guided by special priests; some were led by a ruler who was a sacred figure; some worshiped one god; some, many gods. For all, rituals were a vital part of everyday life.

As part of their worship of nature, gods, and their ancestors, people made rock paintings and fashioned masks, statues, and other objects. Some marked their bodies with dotted lines, spirals, and other shapes—often to indicate the markings of an animal or bird, but always with a special significance. Over the centuries, ritual designs and patterns passed from generation to generation, and the arts flourished and spread through trading networks. Like music and dance, art in its many expressions remains a vital part of African culture.

# EUROPEAN TRADE

BY THE MID-1400S, EUROPEAN TRADE with the African kingdoms was thriving. Led by the Portuguese, Europeans traveled down the west coast of Africa to trade for the riches they found there. Exactly what riches the Europeans sought can be told from the names the Portuguese gave to the regions where they traded.

The Grain Coast, now Liberia, was a fertile agricultural area yielding corn, rice, and other grains. The name, however, does not refer to these grains but to a kind of sweet pepper called *malaguetta*, which means "grains of paradise." This pepper was much sought after in Europe as a seasoning for food.

Below the Grain Coast was the area still called the Ivory Coast, where abundant elephant herds yielded ivory tusks valued all over the world for jewelry and other ornaments. Below the Ivory Coast was the Gold Coast, in the area of present-day Ghana. For two centuries after the Portuguese arrived, in 1471, the Gold Coast was Africa's center of trade with Europe.

A fourth coast was to become an even greater center for trade—the Slave Coast (in present-day Nigeria). Although the name Slave Coast is applied to this one section, slavery became the main trading attraction all along the four-thousand-mile Atlantic coast. To build their colonies and exploit the riches of the New World, the Portuguese and other Europeans took millions of strong young Africans from their homelands.

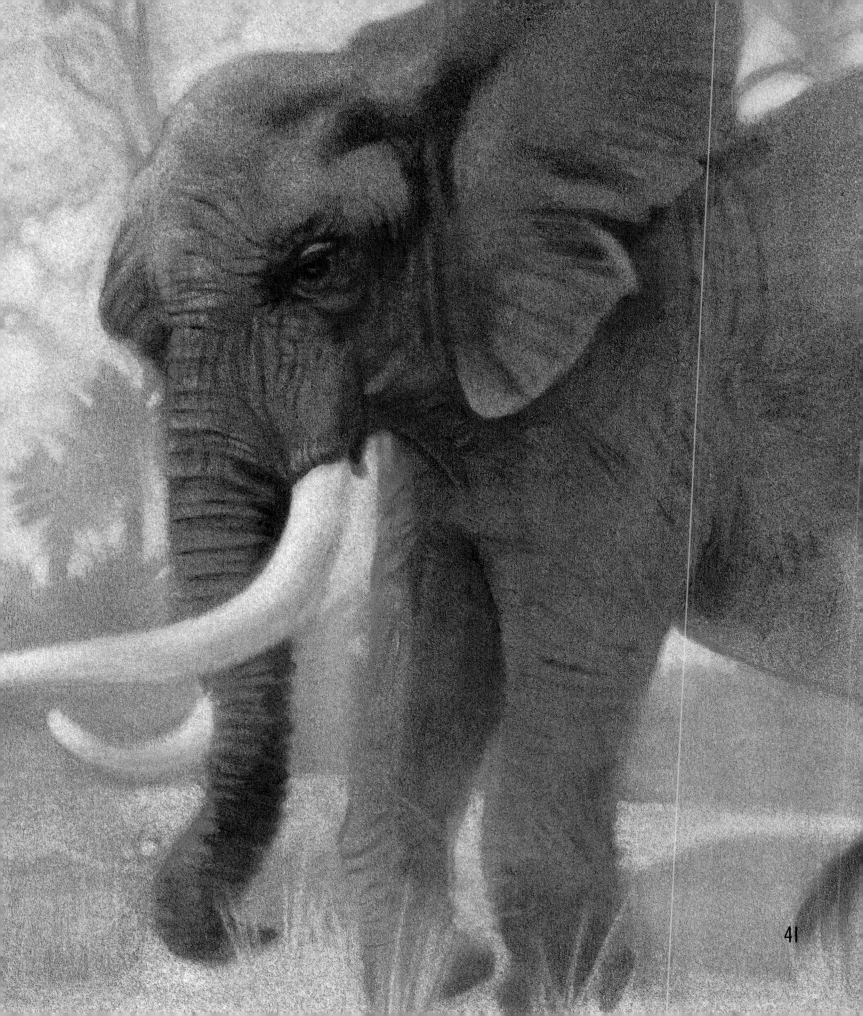

# SLAVERY AND COLONIZATION

SLAVERY HAD LONG EXISTED IN AFRICA, AND A SLAVE TRADE WITH THE ARABS TO THE NORTH HAD BEEN conducted for centuries. Thus, when the Portuguese began taking slaves out of Africa in the 1400s, the African rulers with whom they traded had no objection. In fact, during the years of the organized European slave trade with Africa—from about 1500 to the 1880s, with its peak between 1750 and 1800—many African rulers and entire kingdoms devoted most of their energies to trading in human lives.

In Africa, however, slaves had rights as well as responsibilities. New World slavery was chattel slavery, in which slaves were regarded as property, not people, and had no rights at all. It was a brutal system in which millions died, either on their way to the New World or after they arrived there. During the Middle Passage—the voyage across the Atlantic Ocean—many of the captives committed suicide by jumping overboard or starving themselves rather than be taken to an unknown land and fate. Many more died from the harsh and inhuman conditions on the ships, where they were packed suffocatingly tight into the holds and allowed little fresh air or exercise.

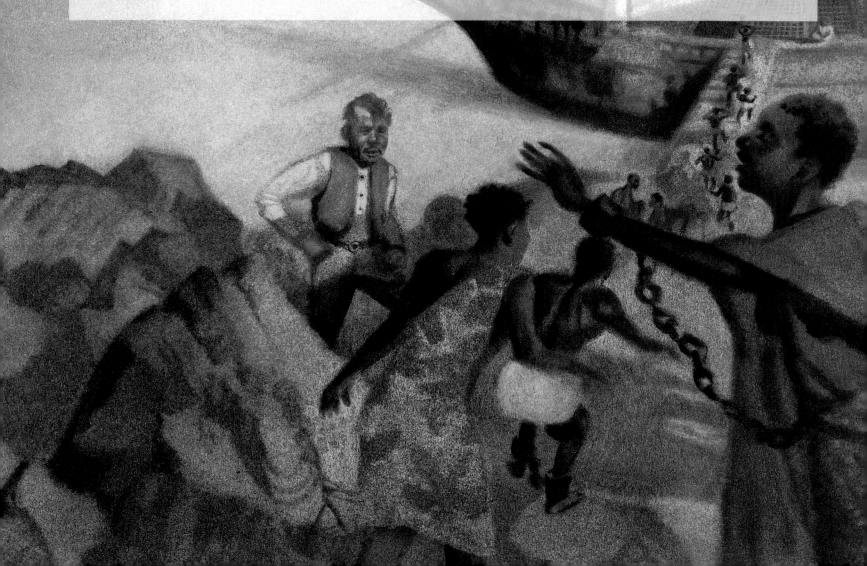

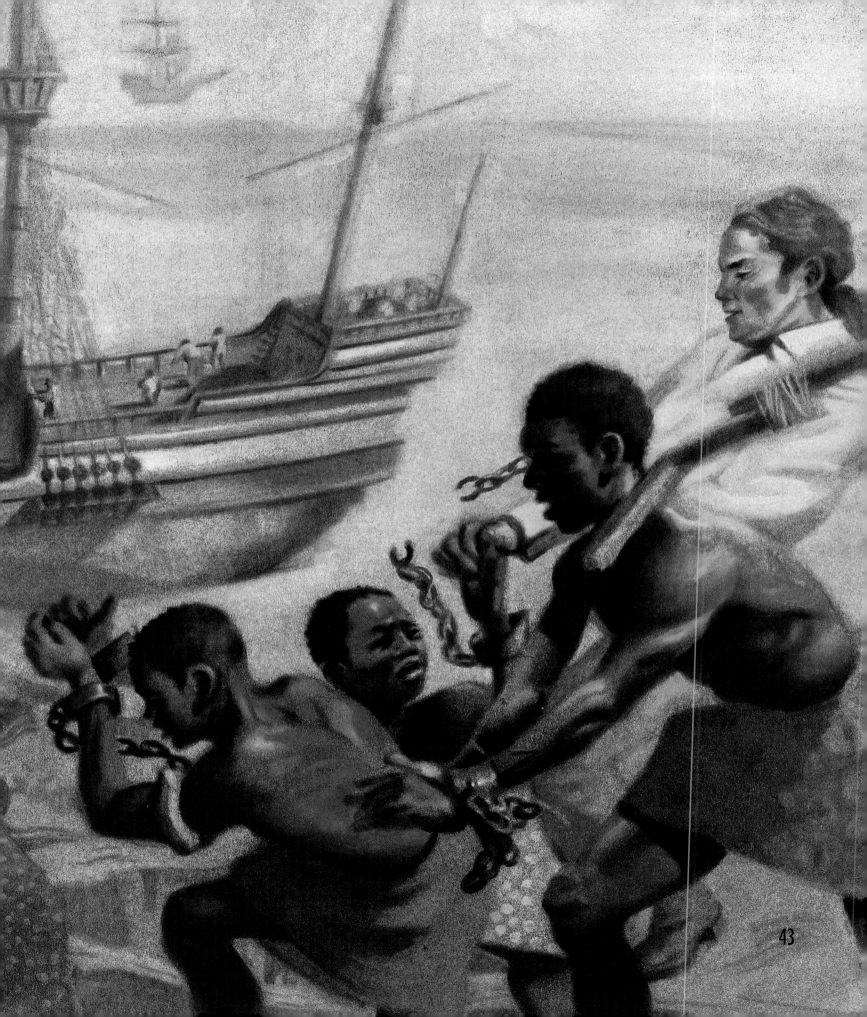

43

Equally great suffering awaited them in the New World, where they were forced to clear forests, dig canals, plant fields, build towns and cities, mine ore and forge iron, raise and shear sheep and weave cloth, tame horses and drive cattle, and care for whole families who were not their own, cooking food and doing laundry, soothing crying babies, healing illnesses, and digging graves—all with little hope of ever escaping their condition.

Not only the slaves themselves suffered. Western Africa as a whole also suffered. Since European traders were eager for Africa's natural resources, economies in Africa became focused on giving up those resources rather than enhancing them through conservation and manufacturing. So many European goods arrived in payment for natural resources and slaves that many African craftsmen, including textile workers and metal processors, stopped making their special products, and many traditions were disrupted. Most important, western Africa suffered from the loss of millions of its youngest, strongest, and healthiest people. Instead of contributing their skills and strengths and intelligence to their homelands, they were forced to use them in the New World.

Yet more sorrow was in store for Africa. Beginning in the late nineteenth century, various European nations colonized the ancient lands, further exploiting the natural resources and the labor of the people. Between 1880 and 1912, all of Africa except Ethiopia and Liberia (colonized by ex-slaves from the United States) fell under the control of European powers. But the peoples of Africa retained their spirit, their strength, and their pride in traditions, and beginning in the early 1950s they threw off the colonial yoke and formed new and independent nations.

So, too, the Africans forcibly taken from their homelands retained their spirit and pride. No one could take their traditions from them, and over the centuries their cultures became part of New World cultures. North, Central, and South American, Caribbean, and West Indian language and literature, music and dance, religion and folklore were all enriched by the influence of slaves. In this way, their African beginnings, though far away and long ago, could never be forgotten.

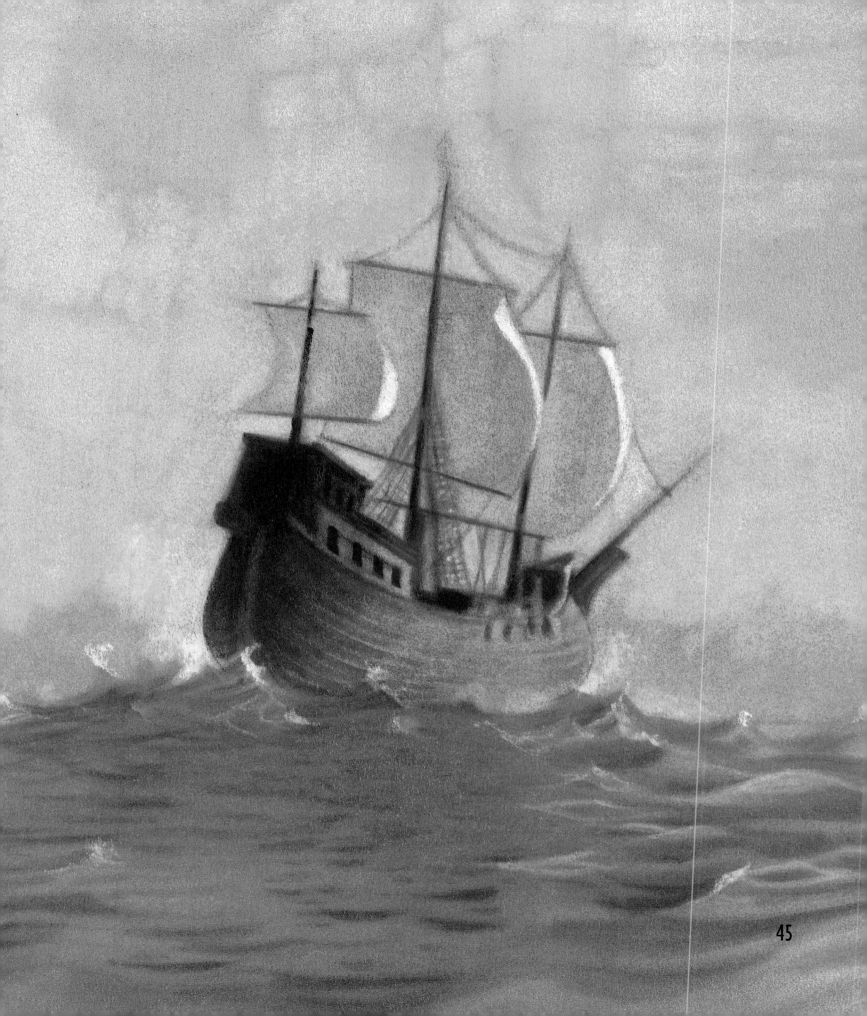

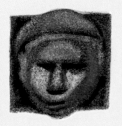

# MILESTONES IN AFRICAN HISTORY

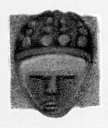

## (MOST DATES ARE APPROXIMATE)

**100,000 B.C.** First *Homo sapiens*, Olduvai Gorge

**35,000** Rudimentary counting devices, South Africa

**24,000** First rock paintings in Africa, Namibia

**7500** Fishing communities in southern Sahara

**6000** Cattle domesticated, Sahara

**5000** Grain farming, Egypt

**3800** Nubian culture begins

**3100** Egypt unifies and system of divine kingship begins

**3000** Egyptians develop writing system

**2650** First Egyptian pyramids built

**2550** Pharaoh Khufu (Cheops) begins pyramids at Giza

**750–650** Kushite kings rule Egypt

**600** Camels introduced to Egypt by Assyrian or Persian invaders

**500** In Nigeria, Nok culture develops; it is to flourish for a thousand years and be the source of the first ironworking in sub-Saharan Africa

**250** Settlement of Jenne-jeno founded as a small farming village

**180** Alphabetic writing appears in Meroë

**100** Meroë, a great industrial center in which iron technology flourishes, at height of power

**51–30** Cleopatra rules Egypt

**A.D. 300–700** Axum (northeastern Ethiopia) a major trading center where gold and bronze coins are minted

**350** Axum conquers Meroë and Christianity is introduced to region

**450–1230** Ghana gold trade flourishes

**600s** Arab traders begin to travel south across the Sahara

**600–700** Bantu-speaking peoples build city of Great Zimbabwe

**800** Rise of West African kingdom of Ghana

**800–1000** Jenne-jeno at height of power

**900** Great Zimbabwe becomes a major power

**1000** Empire of Ghana at its peak, controlling Atlantic ports and trade routes across the Sahara

**1200s** Mandinka people succeed Ghanian rulers

**1240** Sundiata Keita of the kingdom of Kangaba establishes the new empire of Mali, ending the kingdom of Ghana

**1300** Empire of Benin becomes famed for its trade wealth and bronzeworking

**1312–1337** Mansa Musa, Sundiata's grandson, rules Mali and leads his people to convert to Islam; Timbuktu becomes a center of Islamic scholarship

**1324** Mansa Musa travels to Mecca, bringing so much gold with him that there is inflation in the region for many years to come

**1340** Empire of Songhay founded

**1440** Portuguese traders begin taking slaves out of Africa

**1464** Muslim ruler Sonni Ali becomes ruler of Songhay, formerly a province of Mali, and it begins to flourish as a separate empire

**1480–1490** Kingdom of Kongo begins time of significant trade with Portugal

**1493** Songhay empire reaches its greatest height under Askia Muhammad; during his reign, Leo Africanus (a Muslim from Spain) visits Timbuktu and writes that "manuscripts and books are sold for more money than any other merchandise"

**late 1400s** Monomatopan Confederacy ends; Rozwi Confederacy founded; Timbuktu at its height

**1500–1880s** European slave trade with Africa expands to include English, Dutch, and French as well as Portuguese

**1525–1600** Afonso I, ruler of Kongo, controls trade with Europeans and temporarily halts slave trade

**1591** Songhay defeated in Battle of Tondibi; Moroccan occupation lasts until 1618

**1665** Portuguese armies defeat Kongo rulers

**1750–1800** Peak of African slave trade

# BIBLIOGRAPHY

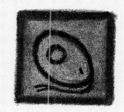

Davidson, Basil. *Africa in History*. Revised and expanded edition. New York: Collier Books, 1991.

————. *African Civilization Revisited: From Antiquity to Modern Times*. Trenton, NJ: Africa World Press, 1991.

————. *The Lost Cities of Africa*. Revised edition. Boston: Little, Brown, 1987.

Everett, Susanne. *History of Slavery*. Secaucus, NJ: Chartwell Books, 1991.

Mazrui, Ali A. *The Africans*. Boston: Little, Brown, 1986.

Oliver, Roland. *The African Experience: Major Themes in African History from Earliest Times to the Present*. New York: HarperCollins, 1992.

Oliver, Roland, and Anthony Atmore. *The African Middle Ages: 1400–1800*. New York: Cambridge University Press, 1989.

Oliver, Roland, and Brian M. Fagan. *Africa in the Iron Age c. 500 B.C. to A.D. 1400*. New York: Cambridge University Press, 1990.

Scarre, Chris. *Smithsonian Timelines of the Ancient World*. New York: Dorling Kindersley, 1993.

Snowden, Frank M., Jr. *Before Color Prejudice: The Ancient View of Blacks*. Cambridge, MA: Harvard University Press, 1991.

## ESPECIALLY FOR YOUNG PEOPLE

Bellerophon staff. *Ancient Africa*. 2 vols. Santa Barbara, CA: Bellerophon Books, 1992–93.

Boyd, Herbert. *African History for Beginners. Part I: African Dawn—A Diasporan View*. New York: Writers and Readers, 1991.

Haskins, James. *Count Your Way Through Africa*. Minneapolis, MN: Carolrhoda Books, 1989.

Haskins, Jim, and Joann Biondi. *From Afar to Zulu: A Dictionary of African Cultures*. New York: Walker, 1995.

Jones, Constance. *Africa, 1500–1900*. New York: Facts on File, 1993.

Mann, Kenny. *Monomatapa, Great Zimbabwe, Zululand, Lesotho: Southern Africa*. Englewood Cliffs, NJ: Silver Burdett, 1996.

McKissack, Patricia C., and Fredrick L. McKissack. *The Royal Kingdoms of Ghana, Mali, and Songhay: Life in Medieval Africa*. New York: Henry Holt, 1995.

Musgrove, Margaret. *Ashanti to Zulu: African Traditions*. New York: Puffin Books, 1992.

# INDEX

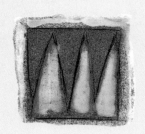
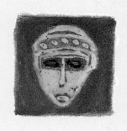

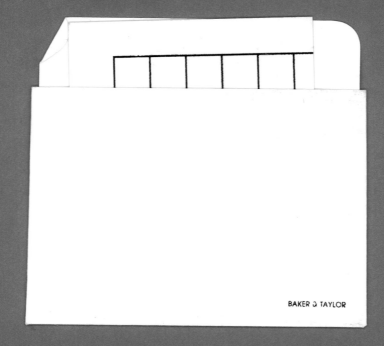

BAKER & TAYLOR